Prais
Take Command Of Your Total Health

As a cheerleader for change for people who are living with the results of poor choices or unfortunate circumstances, Donna is a supportive voice. She was there herself and found the courage to assume responsibility for her own health and happiness, which changed her life. Bravo!!

— Tina Olson

I would definitely recommend this book. So many women over fifty are in a place where we have watched, or are watching, our parents age. Their health is failing and it literally takes a spreadsheet to organize their medications. Every medication has side effects that often times leads to another prescription. I think we are all looking for the kind of advice that the author is providing so we can add more life to our later years and hopefully age more gracefully.

— Michelle Sheehan

Take Command of Your Total Health provides a convincing argument that fifty-plus women can be empowered to live healthier lives. I believe the most persuasive factors were the fact that the author has been on both sides and is living proof that there are many ways to approach your own health care. She has very convincingly shown us that by taking responsibility for your own health both emotionally and physically, you can improve the quality of your life dramatically.

— Michelle Roccia

The author had a convincing argument about Functional Medicine and the positive roll it can play in our modern day health care. I was convinced that it is an avenue to explore with health concerns as well as health maintenance.

— Claudine Clark

The chapter on the author's cancer was probably my favorite and most compelling of the book. I found it very inspiring as well as informative. The chapter left me feeling very optimistic that there are things we all can do to control our destiny and not just sit around hoping to never get a cancer diagnosis.   — Robin Uglietto

Take Command of Your Total Health is not a book to read once. It's a lifestyle reference book to keep and mark up, highlight, mark with sticky notes, copy pages, and file in page protectors—or paste inside cabinet doors.   — Marianne Wronka

Once again, Donna has hit it out of the park! Easy read, it flows from one chapter to another. It is real, honest, and straightforward. Although geared toward fifty-plus women, the info provided is relevant to all ages. Tons of gold nuggets.   — Fran Goldstein

Donna's experience, content, and recipes make the book real. How she has changed her life because of her circumstances makes a convincing argument that we can all do it and should do it.

— Lisa Keohane

Take Command of Your Total Health addresses what every average woman over fifty is looking for. I credit the author for being an inspiration and leading women in the direction of healthy eating. I would recommend this book and encourage women readers to work with Donna for support in creating a healthy way of living.

— Anne Lyon

―――――――――――――

I learned so much from *Take Command of Your Total Health*, the information presented was very useful and easy to read, it was as if Donna was speaking to me. The chapter on bone health and osteoporosis really hit the mark for every woman over fifty, and her recipes are fantastic!

— Mary Sloan

Take Command Of Your Total Health

*A Woman's Guide
to Fearless Aging*

DONNA MARKUSSEN

Take Command of Your Total Health
A Woman's Guide to Fearless Aging
by Donna Markussen

Copyright © 2020 Donna Markussen

The research and information presented in this book is for informational purposes only, and does not take the place of qualified medical care. The content is not intended to be a substitute for professional medical advice, diagnosis, or treatment. Always seek the advice of your physician or other qualified health provider with any questions you may have regarding a medical condition. Never disregard professional medical advice or delay in seeking it because of something you have read in this book.

Published by

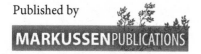

MARKUSSENPUBLICATIONS

ISBN: 978-1-7331036-0-2 (print)
ISBN: 978-1-7331036-1-9 (eBook)
Library of Congress Control Number: 2019913246

Editor: Cynde Christie, WritingCoachCynde.com
Copy editor: Jen Zelinger, TwinOwlsAuthors.com
Book design: Nick Zelinger, NZGraphics.com

First Edition

10 9 8 7 6 5 4 3 2 1

1. Health   2. Nutrition   3. Body, Mind, Spirit

Printed in the United States

This book is dedicated to my husband, Steve, who always believes in me and my vision to serve others in a meaningful way through education and support. Your honesty, wise insights, patience, and sense of humor have profoundly impacted my life in so many ways and have brought me the greatest joy.

To my two sons, Billy and Taylor. Thank you for having such kind hearts and having the courage to own your truth. It is a mother's utmost desire to watch her children blossom through life with confidence, emerging fearlessly to step out of their comfort zone to live life according to their own rules. That is my gift.

To my parents, Mom and Dad, I feel your loving presence every day.

To my in-laws, Mary and Bob, I shall be forever grateful for the love and acceptance you have shown me.

Contents

Preface

To all the women reading this book:

Our bodies are shifting, and we're experiencing hormonal symptoms such as weight gain, low energy, memory issues, hot flashes, or we may have a serious health challenge. All the while, our children have moved on, and we feel our life's purpose has faded into thin air. Now is the time we need to dig deeply to nurture and honor our emotional, physical, and spiritual well-being.

As caregivers, we have always put ourselves last, but not anymore. Wherever you are on your health journey, I hope that this book serves as a bridge between you and a new way of approaching your health and your life. As a mentor and teacher, I would love nothing more than to see you find the confidence to follow your heart, listen to your intuition, and trust that you have it within you to find a better way if what you're currently doing is not serving your well-being. We all want to feel and look sexy, confident, and strong, regardless of what our age is on paper. I hope that you become bold enough to step out of that limiting story to create a new one that enables you to thrive in the next phase of your life!

This was possible for me, and I believe it can be possible for you, too. I had a lifelong struggle with both emotional and physical pain. As you read my story below, it may sound a lot like yours. It may be a different dialogue, but it holds the same universal message.

In my thirties I did not address the issues in my life that weren't working for me: a job I disliked, a schedule that overwhelmed me, and a lack of courage to speak up for myself when I knew I should.

To make matters worse, I was unable to set boundaries, which led to me stuffing away emotions that slowly ate away at my cells. Instead of speaking out or seeking help, I turned to muscle relaxers and pain medications to ease my symptoms. This approach just masked my symptoms, rather than addressing why my symptoms were there in the first place.

Then, at age forty-four, I was diagnosed with breast cancer. Before cancer, I was sleepwalking through my life, not paying any attention to my negative emotions. I was allowing people to overstep their boundaries with me. I'd wake up, go to a job I hated, come home, go to sleep (or at least try), and then do it all over again the next day. This is what I did day after day, week after week, and year after year.

I ignored my desire to want more in life because I believed doing so wasn't a viable option. So, I settled and told myself a story about why my life couldn't change, and I believed this story to be MY truth. I ignored my true inner feelings, and as a result, I always felt pain: emotional pain, back pain, neck pain, headache pain, and stomach pain. I lived this way for years.

I was oblivious to the fact that I was the cause of my own pain and suffering. Slowly, I began to learn that the only way to get out of this madness was to stand up to my pain, and ask, "Why are you here?" I realized I couldn't blame it on my job, my relationships, or my poor health.

I discovered that when you blame external issues like your job, etc., you hand over your power to circumstance, or to the perpetrator who is taking advantage of your well-being, or even to the doctor who is treating your symptoms.

Have you ever found yourself in a similar pattern? If you have, it's time to make a change. Here's how I made mine.

As I continued to go through my discomfort, I grew sick and tired of being sick and tired. That's when I decided to take back control of my personal power. I realized that doctors are not God. I discovered that if you listen, your inner wisdom and intuition would give you the guidance you need to take the next step on your health journey.

Listening to my intuition was a tremendous gift I gave myself. It taught me that I needed to seek additional care to find the root cause of my symptoms. And, when I did, I found Naturopathic and Functional Medicine.

I learned that food is the strongest medication there is, and I changed my diet to reflect a focus on whole foods nutrition. I developed a daily exercise routine, and I took more quality time for myself. I changed the way I perceived my life, which opened me up to a more spiritual practice that placed MYSELF as a priority. This, in turn, gave me more joy without the use of prescription drugs.

You can give this amazing gift to yourself as well. But, it does take time to make this personal investment in yourself. However, I can tell you from my own experience that an investment in your health is the best investment you can make. For me, the time I invested to learn about Functional Medicine saved my life, because Functional Medicine is all about prevention, not just treating symptoms. You deserve this same gift! Here's to the great health you have the power to create!

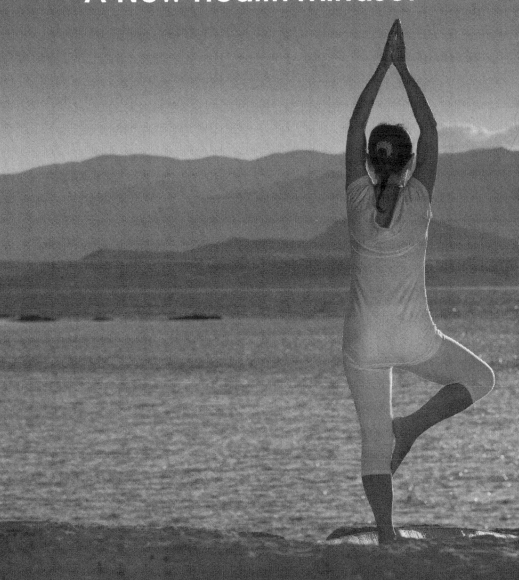

| SECTION 1 |

A New Health Mindset

Introduction

Hi, I'm Donna Markussen, a certified Integrative Nutrition health coach, wife, mother of two wonderful adult boys, and author of *Finding My Way, Facing My Journey With Courage and Notes of Inspiration*. I went from living with chronic neck, shoulder, and back pain, a breast cancer diagnosis at age forty-four, and an autoimmune disease diagnosis that nearly brought me to my knees to living a healthy, vibrant life without the use of medications.

I set out to write this book to target those who are approaching midlife and beyond because we are living within an epidemic of chronic illness and disease, such as heart disease, type 2 diabetes, cancer, autoimmune disease, etc. These diseases are often preventable through early detection and improved diet, exercise, and stress management. Seventy-five percent of people over sixty-five are on various medications, and most of these medications wouldn't be necessary if we understood why our symptoms are there in the first place. For example, sometimes something as simple as cleaning up our diet can dramatically change our health.

Those of us with aging parents are watching them live out their lives tethered to multiple medications, yet still living a poor quality of life. Their generation never questioned the current healthcare model that focuses only on managing symptoms with medications and does not look to the underlying root cause of why those symptoms exist. Their generation wasn't told that the foods you eat have a direct effect on your health.

You don't have to fear your genes. This book's purpose is to let you know that disease and illness do not have to be your fate, even if you're thinking about genetics. I'm a breast cancer survivor, and my mom had breast cancer. Most inherited cases of breast cancer are associated with mutations in two genes: BRCA1 (BReast CAncer gene one) and BRCA2 (BReast CAncer gene two). You inherit one-half of your genes from your mother and one-half from your father. So, if my mother had breast cancer, there's a 50 percent chance I will have it if I carry one of those genes. After going through all of my cancer treatments, I did the genetic testing, and I found out that I did not carry the BRCA1 or the BRCA2 gene mutation. The truth is only 5 to 10 percent of cancer is due to genetics[i]. That means 90 percent of cancer is caused by poor diet, lifestyle, environment, chronic stress, or other factors. My cancer wasn't because my mother had breast cancer. I was under a tremendous amount of chronic stress at the time, due to my limiting beliefs about myself, feelings of unworthiness, and shame. I didn't sleep well, and I ate poorly. It's not your genes but the expression of your genes that determines your health. I explore this more fully in my chapter on cancer.

You must understand that the power is in your hands to choose health, not "*dis-ease.*" I refer to the word *dis-ease* because most of us are not experiencing optimal health. Instead, we're living with chronic ailments, discomfort, low energy, and the like. This type of *dis-ease* has become part of our identity, and we most likely have never thought to address it in a way that will free us from the prison of feeling merely mediocre, as opposed to feeling alive, energized, and well. It's not that we purposefully set out to choose *dis-ease*, it's that we don't understand how the body works and how our daily choices, over an extended period of time, are either feeding into our future ill-health or maintaining and sustaining health as we age. This means your diet, your environment, your lifestyle, your thoughts, and your emotions all play a major role in establishing good health or *dis-ease*. With the study of epigenetics, we learn that our diet, our environment, our lifestyle choices, and our thoughts and emotions strongly influence our gene expression. This means you have the power to turn certain genes on or off, based on what foods you eat, regular exercise, managing stress, cleaning out environmental toxins, and your perception of life. I discuss this in more detail in Chapter 5. This is good news because even if your parents had a certain health issue, you can alter your genetic code now by making the right lifestyle choices.

After reading this book, you'll understand that the third stage of your life can be lived with vitality and health. You'll want to have the energy and strength to do the things that make you feel alive and well. You'll walk away with in-depth knowledge and practical steps to take for nourishing your body, mind, and soul. And know, it's never too late. Our body regenerates itself every day. We have hundreds of thousands of stem cells within our bone marrow and almost all of our organs. These stem cells work as an internal repair system to help regenerate, repair, and maintain our body's health throughout our lifetime.

So, if you're concerned about your aging process, the right foods can help enhance the performance of your stem cells, therefore providing you with the ability to regenerate your body. That means when you eat nourishing foods, your stem cells work to maintain a healthy heart, sharp mind, and strong immune function, heal wounds, and keep your body strong and youthful. It's that simple. The alternative is when we don't take care of our health with a poor diet, we are highly vulnerable to illnesses that attack our bodies throughout our life span.

As we grow older, we have fewer stem cells in our bone marrow. This is why it is vital to maintain those healthy cells as you age. A person with compromised stem cells will know it, as they are living with a chronic disease, such as type 2 diabetes. Stem cells exposed to high sugar environments cannot regenerate and lose their ability to do their job. They can't multiply the way a healthy stem cell can, and thus, lose their ability to help regenerate new tissue. My purpose for sharing this information is so that you can begin transforming your future by implementing the steps outlined in this book today.

You don't have to fear aging when you have the right knowledge to take charge of your health. The old school way of thinking is that when you get older, your health declines and disease is inevitable. It is expected. And when your health declines, you're placed on multiple medications to manage your symptoms, each with their own side effects. It has been etched into our society, the belief that as our health declines there's nothing we can do about it. We're a victim of ill-health and our only hope is managing our symptoms with medication. I'm here to tell you, this does not have to be your fate. When you look at prevention versus just managing your symptoms, you empower yourself to become your own health advocate. When you start to question your old belief system (and other people's belief systems) and look into a more Functional Medicine approach toward your health, you'll feel empowered and understand you have it within you to find health, and not *dis-ease*, as you age.

Listening to your inner doctor is probably the most underutilized healing center available to you. If a medical practitioner is telling you something that doesn't resonate with you, listen to that resistance and explore it. Don't let a doctor tell you it may be (fill in the blanks) and then wear that label, whether you believe it or not. That is called the "nocebo effect." The person with the white coat gives you a diagnosis, and you take on that diagnosis and believe it to be true without investigating it further. But if you want to optimize your chances to reverse your symptoms, you have to start by cleansing your mind of any negative beliefs that will sabotage your healing efforts. You don't have to resign to the prognosis a doctor gives you. This is where research is so important. Get educated on your symptoms and what may be causing them. Seek out a Functional Medicine (or other) health practitioner who can offer you sound advice on looking to the core of your health issue, and take steps to reverse your symptoms or, at the very least, help alleviate them.

A good example of this is when I go to my annual physical, I'm told to get a flu shot. I know this is a personal issue, but I always refuse. Most flu shots have mercury in them, and I question why I would subject my body to a toxic substance like mercury if I don't have to? My point is, I don't subscribe to the fear-based healthcare model and understand that as long as I'm doing the right things, I have a better chance of warding off the flu because I have a healthy immune system. I seek out my inner doctor for advice.

It's important to not subscribe to the it's-all-downhill-from-here attitude. As a society, we are told that as we age, life gets harder, our health declines, and we can't do the things we used to do. We are long overdue for a change in that broken belief system. We need to make a paradigm shift away from "aging equals sickness and ill-health" to "aging equals health, joy, and wellness." Just look at the actress Betty White, who, at the age of 97, working in show business, stated, "I'm blessed with good health. On top of that, I don't go around thinking 'Oh, I'm 97, I better do this, or I better do that.' I'm just Betty. I'm the same Betty that I've always been. Take it or leave it." Growing older takes on a whole new meaning when we approach it knowing we are in control of our health. Instead of spending the last years of your life in poor health, you can have a renewed attitude that will help you flourish physically, emotionally, and spiritually. We have put in our time and have learned a tremendous number of life lessons. Now, we must stand in our power and reject our culture's negative messages about growing older, and instead, make a conscious effort to live life into our sixties, seventies, and eighties with health and wellness, not *dis-ease* and despair.

Now, you're at a crossroads where you get to decide what your life will look like in the years to come. Are you going to grow older with a renewed sense of vitality or grow older with disease and medications? The choice is yours.

The choice I made was to live healthily. I learned that food is the strongest medication there is and changed my diet to reflect whole foods nutrition, daily exercise, and taking more quality time for myself. I changed the way I perceived my life, which opened me up to a more spiritual practice where I placed myself as a priority, which in turn, gave me more joy without the use of prescription drugs. What an amazing gift you can give yourself. However, it does take time to invest in yourself this way.

You will read a lot about Functional Medicine in this book because it is all about *prevention*, not just treating symptoms. While I admire and respect our conventional medicine when treating trauma, cancer therapies, acute illnesses, and using cutting-edge therapies and medications that save lives, etc., they don't help you to understand that most illnesses take years to manifest, and what you do behind the scenes in those years (diet, lifestyle, exercise, stress, and environment) become your building blocks to either health or ill-health later on. If you can understand this important concept, that food is your best medicine, and you can recognize the importance of fueling your body instead of depleting it, it can help you avoid a diagnosis of chronic illness later on in life. It's time to start taking care of yourself physically, mentally, emotionally, and spiritually. It is my hope that after reading this book, you'll have a better understanding of the steps you can take now to prevent disease later on or, at the very least, add in some holistic treatments in addition to what you are doing to help yourself feel whole again.

When I was able to get to the root cause of my symptoms, it changed my life. I now have energy, vitality, and joy. Here are some of the things that I can now enjoy regularly:

- Hot yoga and Pilates classes three to four times a week
- Daily long walks with my dog
- Hiking in the mountains of New Hampshire
- Resistance training and HIIT twice a week
- Peloton rides
- Taking the stairs instead of the elevator whenever I want
- Understanding what foods are causing inflammation in my body
- Setting clear boundaries when I feel it is necessary, without guilt
- Challenging myself with new projects, always learning and growing

What will be on your list?

It is my wish to help you achieve your health goals. Just for reading this book, I would like to give you a free gift. Go to *https://www.donnamarkussen.com.*

CHAPTER 1

Reframing Your Story

"Guilt is that feeling we run from when we see it coming, yet we can't seem to hide. Guilt is a major happiness robber. Guilt takes up valuable real estate in our mind and tricks us into thinking we are wrong and the perpetrator is right. Guilt plays with our self-esteem and keeps us in the victim mentality, prohibiting our ability to find the true picture of what is really happening. And, by the way, when we befriend guilt, it means the person who is robbing our energy wins!"

Our life's journey is uniquely our own, and for most of us, we feel as if we are damaged goods. You may be suffering from a health challenge that contributes to your sadness or worries about your future. What is your story around your health? Do you live with optimism or fear? Can you open your mind up to look at this challenge as a way for you to explore your feelings more and see how they are sabotaging your well-being? You can just as easily create a new story that will introduce you to a better version of yourself and break free from the fear narrative you're currently holding on to. You can reframe your story in a way that empowers you to learn and grow from each circumstance or struggle that you encounter. A new concept? Maybe, but the alternative is staying in a disempowering state of despair and not finding a better path that will lead you to new answers and support. Know that your health challenge has meaning behind it, and you need to take a deeper look at your thoughts, emotions, lifestyle choices, and limiting beliefs about yourself. How are you spending your free time? Are you catering to everyone else's needs and not your own? You may feel trapped in a life that doesn't align with your heart and soul. And when you're not taking care of yourself or setting clear boundaries to protect your own well-being, you're putting everyone else's health and welfare ahead of your own. Who is going to take care of your needs if you don't?

In my first book, *Finding My Way*, I wrote about how I learned from the many health challenges I went through and the story (feeling unworthy) I had told myself that held me hostage. The book's purpose was to show others, by example, the importance of owning and learning from our own challenges in life. I was able to break free from the emotional self-sabotage that caused me a ton of physical and emotional pain. This process of self-discovery led me to find the courage to explore my emotions and limiting beliefs about myself, which helped me to break the habit of self-sabotage.

When we look back at our lives, what story are we telling? We are living in a society that has so much noise. We are constantly sifting through all of that noise, picking out the narrative that makes the most sense in our circumstances. This happens most when hit with a diagnosis. Then we receive a prognosis or a typical course of action, and we settle for it. However, what if the story we choose prohibits us from gaining a broader perspective? You may be confused about a recent diagnosis and fear the unknown. Now you get to pick the narrative that makes the most sense. And because it's human nature to default to the negative narrative first, we settle into our victim story instead of looking for answers outside of what our current doctors or situations are telling us. When we face our journey with courage, we have faith that "everything that is happening is *for* me instead of happening *to* me."

It is human nature to see the negative before we can see the positive. It's becoming aware of our human, natural default mechanisms that enable us to change. When we fall prey to those negative assumptions, we don't have the ability to choose a different path. There is always a different path; we just need to explore more.

Our stories reflect back to us how we perceive life. Two people could go through the same situation, and both would have a different narrative (story) based on their world, which consists of their thoughts, beliefs, and perceptions. When our story is working against us, we can just as easily change that narrative to reflect how we want to live.

In the workbook section of *Finding My Way, Facing My Journey with Courage*, I wrote:

> Some of the most profound life lessons learned are from the many struggles endured during our journey, including those horrific life events such as an illness, the loss of a loved one, losing a job, challenging financial situations, or a child dangerously succumbing to drugs or alcohol. We get to choose how we deal with each situation. Instead of hitting the pause button and replaying our story repeatedly, while gaining a powerful vortex-like momentum of victimhood, we hit the delete button and begin a new story, one that is full of optimism, hope, courage, and strength. By staying focused on our goal, the result we desire, we choose a better way.

Kim Schneider, in *Step Out of Your Story*, stated:

> With imagination and well-directed self-inquiry, we can step out of our story, check out the landscape, and determine whether to stay on our current path or to go in a different direction. We can then transform obstacles into opportunities to break bad habits and improve our character to become the real hero of our own living, evolving story.

In *Finding My Way*, I also talk about my own personal boundary challenges. When I stood up for myself, I became a much happier person. I wrote:

> If we don't honor ourselves by setting clear boundaries, we remain the main character in our victim story, letting others dictate how we move through life. When we ignore our own feelings, we are putting other people's health and welfare ahead of our own.

You deserve to feel good.

You deserve to protect yourself from people and things that make you feel bad.

You deserve to honor all that is inside of you.

By mindfully taking care of ourselves, we will be available for others in a more meaningful way. In order for us to put our world in order, we must first cultivate our own lives, take the steps to fuel our body and practice self-care, and know where our heart lies. That's when we can begin to help others see their light.

Some of us self-sabotage our health and use food to improve our mood. Instead of facing our feelings and emotions, we turn to a pint of ice cream, a large pizza, or some other food indulgence after a rough day. Then we're left with feelings of guilt. It's time to ditch the guilt and figure out what's causing you to feel this way. When we have the awareness to deal with an issue instead of hiding from it, we'll break ourselves free from emotional self-sabotage and get our health back.

Understand that treating yourself occasionally is normal behavior; there is nothing wrong with celebrating. On the other hand, using food to quell unhappy feelings or to fill a void is a problem. Doing so may cause a momentary sense of relief, but it ultimately brings more negative emotions than good ones. The guilt and shame can send us down a spiral that, in turn, can cause more emotional eating, thereby creating a cycle of behavior that is difficult to stop.

If this has been happening to you often, it's time to dig a little deeper, see what's going on underneath the surface, and find new tools to defeat the habit.

Let's touch on some ways you can create new patterns without guilt:

1. **Feel your feelings.** Staying with your feelings, no matter how uncomfortable, is essential for battling emotional eating. It's ok to feel your feelings; embrace them instead of making the decision to avoid them. The sooner you acknowledge those feelings, the sooner they will disappear. Write about them in a journal and release them. Talk them through with a friend or loved one. Reserve your tasty treats for your chosen special days, not for when your emotions are driving you to them.

2. **Savor the moment.** Look for the moments in your life that are lighthearted and happy. The clouds in the sky, the way the sun feels on your face, a relaxing bubble bath ... these are all things to savor. Do it with your food as well, and eat mindfully. Enjoy that slice of veggie pizza, but take each bite with thoughtfulness and honestly eat for enjoyment, not to snuff out feelings.

3. **Don't eat unless you're hungry.** Make sure you're hungry before you eat. If you aren't sure, have a glass of water first. Wait ten minutes after drinking it, and if you still feel hungry, now's the perfect time to reach for a bite to eat. Exercise healthy eating 80 percent of the time, and when you mindfully and moderately indulge, it will have less of an impact. Balance is everything, and I live by this myself too!

4. **Know your triggers.** Keeping a journal will help you see what triggers set you off for emotional eating. When you identify what makes you head for the fridge, then you can stop those triggers in their tracks.

5. **Keep healthy in your control.** Get the enemy out of your house! It's easy to be tempted to reach for that bowl of ice cream when it's stored in your freezer! Stock your fridge with delicious yet nutritious foods so that the temptation isn't there. Carrot sticks with hummus is a satisfying snack that takes little to no effort to prepare. When you make healthier choices all around, it's easier to control your emotional eating.

| CHAPTER 2 |

Wonder Woman Syndrome

"No one can fix your life for you. You need to set out consciously to do it for yourself. You must trust what you know in your bones—that your body is your ally and that it will always point you in the direction you need to go next."
— Christiane Northrop, MD

I want you to take a good look at your energy levels. Do you feel energized or depleted on most days? Maybe you never really thought about assessing how you are feeling. Most women have maternal instincts and default to being the almighty caregiver for their loved ones, even at their own expense. Whether that's providing for your aging parents or children, responsibilities at work, and other obligations, you forget to address your own health and your own aging process. Deep down, you feel you should have it all together, sitting back and enjoying the ride from all your fruitful years of working diligently, raising kids, managing schedules, etc. After all, it's supposed to be the time in your life for you to reap the rewards of all your hard work. You even have the wisdom and experience to know that eating organic, non-GMO foods are good for you and make a conscious effort to do so. Still, you keep experiencing an underlying feeling of malaise. What is it? Well, it may be one of the most misdiagnosed illnesses out there. There isn't a doctor on the planet who will tell you this information. No blood test will show you what's going on. The only way to address your symptoms head-on is to ask yourself, "What am I doing that is making me feel this way?"

For those of us sandwiched between the escalating needs of our aging parents and kids who haven't quite figured out their lives, we're stuck in an intergenerational squeeze. We feel we must take care of every problem that comes our way. We live our lives like Wonder Woman, that almighty superwoman who can take on anything because she has the power and strength to do so. She keeps going, keeps fighting, keeps doing, keeps providing because that's her job. How many of us live our lives this way?

Let's take a step back and look at the big picture. We will use our older children as an example. To become adults, our children need to learn, grow, stumble, make mistakes, and face their fears. However, if we are constantly doing, deciding, and providing, we are not allowing them to know, with conviction, their own truth. And, while our intentions are good, they will never know their own strengths and weaknesses. If we go through life carrying them on our backs, we're also putting a tremendous burden on ourselves. More importantly, how does that serve them in their world? How do they learn to get the courage to speak up to a boss when they feel, deep down, they may be wrong? There will be times in their lives that they will need to stand up and question authority. If they don't have the skill set to do so, they will remain silent. That silence will follow them all through their lives, and they won't have the confidence to take a stand for themselves because they won't know, deep down, who they are.

When we take on the world's problems, we can't address our own needs. When we ignore our feelings, we cause stress. This type of silent stress causes both emotional and physical pain. A doctor does not diagnose this type of stress. This stress is not tangible stress, like being in an unhappy relationship or job you dislike. You won't identify it as stress because it has become your identity. You have surrendered to it. However, understand, when we withhold from ourselves, we are withholding from others as well. Wouldn't you rather be an example of what you want your children to become? If we are not allowing our children to grow, we are not growing. The greatest gift you can give yourself is growth. Be the example you want for your children, and they will want to become that person. It certainly beats lecturing them. We all know how that turns out. Allow them to learn, grow, and stumble as much as possible. You will be their emotional support system, but allow them to live the experience of life.

You may be thinking, "How can I not help the people I love?" There will be times when it makes perfect sense to step in and help out, but when it becomes habitual and your loved ones are relying on you, that's when you know this enabling has to stop. You are not serving your loved ones by enabling them. On the contrary, you are *disabling* them by preventing them from learning the problem-solving skills they will need to maneuver through a complicated life. If you can make a paradigm shift in your beliefs to see the truth in this, you will think twice about giving up your valuable time to take care of their issues.

You may be thinking that this will only create more stress and cause you more anxiety. Try to reverse that thought and know that you are serving them in a major way by allowing them to practice their life skills, while still being there for moral support. Then you will have peace.

The first step is to understand that you need to unlearn your prior beliefs and behaviors that are prohibiting you from seeing the big picture. Our deepest beliefs and assumptions will determine if we stay present and open to shining a new light on a situation—or remain the same and let our old habits control us. You take on their world; however, if that world is not serving your well-being, how does that work? How much longer do you continue on this path, until you're hit with a wake-up call in the form of *dis-ease,* depression, or despair? What if you could learn to set a clear intention—*I deserve more—*

more *joy*, more *peace*, more *happiness*, and more *time for myself*. I know if you had a best friend who was distraught and caught in a similar situation, you would advise him or her to let go and take care of themselves before they became sick. When we live this intentional way, we demonstrate to others by example how important it is to respect our self-care and ourselves.

To understand our hidden beliefs and assumptions, we need to rewind those tapes of our lives to unravel when and why we acquired those beliefs in the first place. Those beliefs come from fear. If we fear rejection or disapproval, we feel unworthy to speak up when we know we should. This sends the message that it isn't safe to disagree with others. Most likely, we learned this thinking from our parents, grandparents, and others in our early life environment. I can empathize with this because this was me!

Consequently, we don't recognize our beliefs as a problem because they are all we know. However, when we find the courage to observe those limiting beliefs at arm's length and change them according to our *intentions*, we will gain the *courage* to change, knowing it is in everyone's best interest for us to do so. Trusting yourself this way takes practice.

Ask yourself, "How does it feel to slow down, step back, disengage, and prioritize self-care?" It may feel awkward at first, as we are living in a culture that does not value self-care. This is why it is important to make a conscious shift in your core beliefs. You deserve to take care of yourself this way. You deserve to live your third phase of life nourishing your mental, physical, and spiritual well-being to ensure health, not *dis-ease*, as you age.

When we take care of ourselves this way, we age gracefully. Age is a number, but how you age is definitely your choice. And the things you do every day will determine how fast you age. Just go to any power yoga class, and you can find women and men into their sixties and seventies participating in yoga poses, standing in their power and feeling strong. I look up to people such as that because I realize they didn't let society influence them. They understand they are responsible for taking care of their bodies, and no antiaging cream, fad diet, or miracle drug is going to cultivate self-worth and self-esteem, and in the same way, doing what they do on a daily basis intentionally nurtures their bodies, minds, and souls.

Everywhere you look, you see commercials on antiaging. There are billions of marketing dollars promoting antiaging products for women and men, and many people are eager to purchase anything that will help slow down their biological clocks. While I'm all for the nourishing and hydrating creams that help us keep a youthful glow, sometimes we're missing the bigger picture of what ages us.

Most of us, moving into our midlife and beyond, have more of a handle on how we want to live out the third phase of our life, as we've lived and learned from the past mistakes we made along the way. However, what happens if you're still stuck in the overcommitted, frantic schedule or a less-than-ideal work life and you're busy managing your adult children's lives? Because you're so busy, you do not take the time to eat a healthy diet or take care of your body. You can't seem to find the time to take care of yourself and do the things that will feed your soul and body. Instead, you're letting *life lead you*, and deep down, you know there has to be a better way.

One of my favorite quotes from the late Wayne Dyer is: "When you change the way you look at things, the things you look at change."

When *we change the way we look at things*, we can reroute our old thinking patterns toward a more intentional way of living. Think of what a TV remote control does. You pick it up, and you change the channels to search for a program you want to watch. You're in control; the TV won't change channels on its own. In a sense, when you're not intentionally taking care of yourself, feeding your body with nutrient-dense foods, doing physical exercise to stay strong, and setting clear boundaries, you're giving away your remote to circumstances that will dictate how you move through your life. You're not in control; the situation at hand is pushing the buttons of your remote.

You must understand that managing your health and your mental well-being is your job, and your daily job description is not to allow negative outside circumstances in that don't serve you. When we don't address the things in our life that are not working, it promotes chronic feelings of anger and resentment. These toxic emotions will change the way your genes get expressed and accelerate the aging process. Mainstream medicine does not address this, and instead, they'll offer you something to help with your anxiety and emotions with medication. These toxic feelings can cause a lifelong, bitter battle with yourself and increase your stress levels, causing your immune system to suffer. Ask yourself, "Who has the remote to my life?" Is it you, the circumstance, or a perpetrator whom you feel has wronged you?

Asking for help, whether it's from a family member, friend, or a professional outside supporter will help you find time to take care of yourself as you move through your own aging process. The more self-aware you are when a situation outside of your control is not serving you, the easier it is for you to take steps and ask for help, without the guilt. When you do, you can focus on the things that bring you joy, instead of just wallowing in those negative feelings of resentment, anger, and despair.

When you take care of yourself this way, you no longer give your remote away to others, you slow down the aging process, and your self-confidence soars. My next chapter delves further into taking control of your emotional pain and shows how *that* can be the driver of your physical pain or illness.

CHAPTER 3

Healing from Emotional Wounds and Past Trauma

In this chapter, I want to introduce you to how powerful your thoughts, beliefs, and emotions can be and how they have a huge impact on your health. For some of you, the information shared here may be somewhat new, and if so, it is my hope that you gain valuable knowledge about the mind-body connection. You can shave years off your suffering when you understand this information and take additional steps to improve your overall health condition.

We are conditioned to believe that someone other than ourselves knows more about our bodies than we do. But what if we looked at our symptoms, such as a skin rash, pain in our joints, low energy, back pain, neck pain, headache, etc., as our body's way of giving us feedback that there's an imbalance in our life somewhere? Your body is constantly trying to talk to you. This is when intuition plays a key role as your interpreter to help you understand that you need to investigate why these things are happening. Learn the language of intuition, and you'll start to feel more confident about how to proceed.

Our body's design promotes healing, and in fact, healing is happening every moment. For example, when we have inflammation, it is a healing response of our body trying to get back into balance. However, when we are overloaded with inflammation, our body is unable to complete its primary function.

When we're diagnosed with chronic pain and other ailments, we feel as though our bodies are working against us. But when we're hit with some form of *dis-ease* or discomfort, it's a sign we must change our focus on what is taking our time and attention away from those issues in our life we need to address in order to heal. This happens when we realize our emotional, physical, and spiritual healing begins when we become aware of where we are directing our attention (negative thoughts), we begin removing the people and circumstances that don't serve our well-being (boundaries), we address our past emotional trauma, and we stop neglecting our body with a poor diet and sedentary lifestyle.

Your symptoms are uniquely yours, and you can heal them with the right mindset, tools, education, and support. The power of thought alone can heal you when you believe it is possible. Your mind can become a powerful healing tool when used the right way. You may be familiar with the placebo effect. Most drug studies use placebos. There are two groups of people seeking treatment for a specific condition. The first group takes the actual drug, while the second group receives a sugar pill, or placebo, although they do not know that what they are taking is not the real thing.

These clinical trials help researchers measure if a drug works by comparing how both groups react. If both groups have the same reaction, whether they see improvements or not, the drug is not considered effective. The key here is that those in the placebo group with positive reactions *believed* they were taking the real pill and responded positively to treatment. A connection in the brain turns on the healing response. Professor Ted Kaptchuk of Harvard Affiliated Beth Israel Deaconess Medical Center (whose research focuses on the placebo effect) states, "The placebo effect is more than positive thinking, believing a treatment or procedure will work. It's about creating a stronger connection between the brain and body and how they work together."

When symptoms arise, our approach is often to seek medical advice. While it's important to do this step to rule out an organic issue, in the conventional medical world, a doctor will share his or her opinion and throw out some statistics, based on their experience, and give you a diagnosis. Then you get a prognosis. Yet, the original reason remains unaddressed. Emotional and physical pain will not go away on its own. To heal, you have to believe there is something more you can do to alleviate your symptoms and improve your condition.

This concept can be a scary place to land because for most of us, we're dealing with past trauma that we may have been holding on to since childhood. And we taught ourselves that it is "safe to be quiet" and just move on to feel better. Whether it was dealing with an alcoholic parent or physical and emotional abuse from a family member, spouse, etc., until we can bring these deep-rooted emotions to the surface, we cannot heal them. What we don't realize is past trauma, if not addressed, follows you throughout your entire life. It gets triggered by situations that arise, that remind you of those old feelings and emotions stored deeply in your subconscious that you may not even realize are there.

I know because this was me. I used to abuse my own body by contracting my muscles so tightly, I caused myself headaches, back-aches, neck pain, etc. This was my memory response as a little girl when I watched my mother lose control, yelling, screaming, slamming doors, and throwing things, causing me a tremendous amount of fear and anxiety. I wasn't able to release those fears and emotions until much later in life (in my late forties) when I began doing my post-cancer self-discovery work. I am grateful to have had so many healing practitioners to help me move through that process and now understand why I was in so much pain. I forgave, accepted, and loved my mother and realized she was dealing with her own demons and did the best she could at the time. That realization helped me move on with my life.

Find the courage to seek new answers. Courage is a muscle that, with practice, you can build upon. When we're sick or in pain, the unknown can be scary. When our body is not doing so well, we tend to default to the worst-case scenario, and we reach for the negative thoughts and go deeper into despair. That's where self-awareness plays a pivotal role in our healing process. Think about the language that you use to talk to yourself. We default to negative thoughts. However, through self-awareness and self-nurture, you can just as easily switch directions into positive thoughts so that you can begin your healing journey.

The healing process works like this: You want to allow yourself to feel what you're feeling but not wallow in it and discuss it with outside friends and family, who will only help you build upon your grief, even though they mean well. Allowing yourself to feel overwhelmed, scared, confused, and angry for a short period of time is part of the process. The key is not to stay in that vortex. This will work against you and suppress your immune function.

When we're not feeling well, over time, we begin to judge ourselves and think, "There's something wrong with me," which only causes more pain and suffering. And we'll find proof that our judgment is right. Whatever we focus on expands. When we're focusing on how bad we feel, we feel worse.

Look at those feelings of negativity and frustration as something that has crossed your path and is now inviting you to find the message. Ask yourself, "Why am I feeling this way? What am I not seeing?" The more you ignore your feelings, the louder the emotion gets and the worse the pain sets in.

Negative emotions surface like this:

- Anger
- Sadness
- Fear/anxiety
- Shame
- Guilt

- Rage
- Jealousy

Putting your body into a stress response that creates inflammation and other detrimental effects sets the stage for not only physical pain but also for other chronic illnesses. All of the emotions above can be misleading. You may be feeling angry or sad, but at its core lies a deep-rooted emotion, often suppressed for months, years, or sometimes decades. Some of us learned during childhood to ignore bad feelings, or our parents told us to stop complaining and just "be nice." This leads to emotional avoidance, and when we avoid our emotions, we abuse ourselves through addiction, emotional eating, negative self-talk, etc.

Positive emotions are:

- Love
- Kindness
- Joy
- Compassion
- Acceptance

Positive emotions release healing hormones and neurochemicals like oxytocin, serotonin, and dopamine. It's empowering to know that when negative emotions arise, you can become aware of them, acknowledge them, and release them, then pivot to focus on gratitude or something else that cultivates joy for you. Take a few minutes out of your day to remember everything for which you are grateful. Write in your journal your true wins for that day. This simple yet highly effective practice will shift your focus. It's a moment-by-moment choice.

When you come from a place of believing that everything in your life is serving you, then you know that this experience is helping you find your whole self again. Going through this process can be a challenge, but the more you resist it, the harder it will be to heal. When you can express your feelings, acknowledge them, and then try to understand what the message is in this experience, you begin your self-discovery process. This is when you begin to take back control of your life. You take steps to educate yourself and surround yourself with the right people instead of listening to the negative statistics from your doctor, friends, and family about your condition. Remember, holding in your emotions can lead to physical disease later on. So, as I mentioned earlier, don't stay in victimhood for too long.

There is a gift in every challenge. Our job is to educate ourselves so we can find ourselves again. Trauma, chronic stress, and negative emotions all play a key role in us getting sick, and they will continually knock on our door until we face them.

There are therapies available to you that will help you process your pain, in order to heal. These therapies will help you work through trauma, chronic stress, and negative emotions. These emotions can be complex and vary from person to person. But my experience has been to find those alternative healing practitioners who can help you *process* your pain. You may understand your pain intellectually but to get to the subconscious core, you have to pull that pain to the surface and face it head-on. This opens the wound, and it's scary and uncomfortable. Our survival mechanism wants to bury our old wounds, so we numb ourselves by hiding them.

Many avenues are available to you to help resolve past trauma, including finding a good hypnotherapist, therapist, life coach, energy healer, reiki master, craniosacral therapist, emotional freedom technique (EFT) practitioner, tension and trauma release exercises (TRE®) practitioner, or other healing service provider who will help release past trauma, negative emotions, and energy that blocks your system. This type of pain is very hard to process on your own; you need to peel back the onion in order to start to heal.

There is a wonderful documentary on this subject called *HEAL*. I would highly recommend watching this movie, as it offers in-depth conversations with patients who have healed from various traumas and illnesses and reveals how the latest science shows we are not victims of unchangeable genes, nor should we buy into a scary diagnosis. The movie highlights the fact that we have more control over our health and lives than we know we do. This film will empower you with a new understanding of the miraculous nature of the human body and the extraordinary healer within us all. Through many inspiring and emotional stories, we find out what works, what doesn't, and why. Go to *http://www.healdocumentary.com.* [ii]

CHAPTER 4

What Conventional Medicine Is Not Telling You

One of my favorite Functional Medicine practitioners I follow is Chris Kresser. Chris teaches and practices Functional Medicine. In contrast to conventional medicine, which focuses on treating and suppressing symptoms with medication or surgery, Functional Medicine takes a more personalized approach. It addresses the whole person, not just an isolated set of symptoms. In addition, Functional Medicine focuses on shifting the traditional disease-centered medicine to a more patient-centered approach to help eliminate symptoms by addressing the root of the problem and identifying the diet, lifestyle, and environmental factors that cause disease.

In his new book, *Unconventional Medicine: Join The Revolution to Reinvent Healthcare, Reverse Chronic Disease, and Create a Practice You Love*, Chris writes, "Chronic disease is a slow-motion plaque that is sabotaging our health, destroying our quality of life, shortening our lifespan, bankrupting our governments, and threatening the health of future generations."

His book's message highlights the broken model of conventional medicine when treating chronic illness and serves to educate and inform healthcare professionals to shift their focus away from the Band-Aid approach of treating disease with medications toward a healthy whole foods nutrition approach, mind-body practices, exercise, and self-care. His private practice includes Functional Medicine practitioners, nurse practitioners trained in Functional Medicine, physician assistants, nutritionists, health coaches, and services such as acupuncture, physical therapy, occupational therapy, and more that complement his methods. It is my hope that more alternative and Functional Medicine practitioners follow this healthcare model. It would be easier for the patient, less costly, and we would see a greater success rate at overcoming chronic illness.

Many wonderful Functional Medicine and Naturopathic doctors out there have the training to get to the root cause of your problem, not just treat the symptoms. They believe food is medicine, food *is* powerful.

An increasing amount of research in the study of epigenetics demonstrates the effectiveness of lifestyle interventions and whole foods nutrition for the treatment of chronic disease. One's nutritional status also contributes to gene expression. So, if you're eating foods that don't agree with you, loaded with excessive sugar, white flour, gluten, processed foods, GMOs, pesticides and herbicides, artificial ingredients, etc., you're headed toward disease.

Functional Medicine is all about *prevention*, not just treating symptoms. Another good thing is that you gain valuable knowledge as you work with your doctor. That knowledge will stay with you for the rest of your life. As a health coach, I see a lot of confusion about which treatment is best for a particular symptom. With Functional Medicine, the answer is that everyone is unique, and we all come with a bio-individual set of needs. Just like there is no one-diet-fits-all, there is no single approach to treating disease either. Functional Medicine doctors work with the individual as a whole to uncover the underlying root cause of their symptoms and then make recommendations such as changes in diet, lifestyle, and environment to improve and sometimes reverse the patient's overall condition, often without the need to stay on medication, whereas conventional medicine focuses on managing and treating symptoms after they have already occurred. They take a more generalized approach to suppress symptoms with medication, and therefore, the patient relies on medication for the rest of their life, often living with many side effects. This approach doesn't cure their disease; it only manages it to the degree their body responds to the medication.

If there is one thing I've learned on my health journey, it is the importance of taking my health into my own hands. In other words, it's up to me to seek the right care if I don't feel well served by the care that I'm currently receiving. The first step is to declare that you have it within you to seek additional care if what you presently are receiving isn't working for you. Your health and happiness deserve your full attention.

The standard American diet (SAD) is contributing to chronic *dis-ease*, so much so that chronic disease seems normal; it's inevitable. We're not addressing the reality of the SAD diet, which consists of conventional red meat, processed deli meat, conventional poultry (fed antibiotics), processed food products, fried foods, refined grains, genetically modified corn, and soy, and excessive intake of white flour and sugar, processed breads, sugary beverages, and hydrogenated oils, all leading to a pro-inflammatory, low-nutrient, high-calorie disaster. Eating this way plants the seed of disease. Just ask the patient that walks into her doctor's office with her lab work, and it shows that she is pre-diabetic. She's told to keep an eye on it, and when she comes back with the full-blown disease, her doctor will then treat her symptoms. My question is, "Why wait for disease to happen?" With the knowledge that *food is medicine*, we can focus on reversing and preventing chronic disease, rather than managing it.

The Study of Epigenetics

When we have this knowledge, we can control how our genes get expressed. We are living within a global epidemic of chronic disease. Aging baby boomers are living longer but have higher rates of chronic disease, more disability, and lower health compared with the previous generation. The sad truth is it's not just baby boomers getting sicker; our children are getting sicker as well. According to a 2013 report by the National Research Council and Institute of Medicine (NAC/IOM), this shocking statistic is very real. "Americans have been dying at younger ages than people in almost all other high-income countries."[iii]

According to the Centers for Disease Control and Prevention, the United States spends significantly more money on health care than any other country in the world. Seventy-five percent of those dollars are going toward aiding people with chronic conditions.[iv]

We treat our symptoms with medication and surgery but don't look at the root cause. As a nation, we are sicker for a number of reasons. One of the major reasons is that we are eating poorly and feeding our kids highly processed junk food. The food industry knows how to make a food product addictive, which makes you crave more of a bad thing. We are eating fast food on the run with our busy lifestyles; then we're living with chronic stress 24-7.

Can lifestyle choices affect our gene expression? The answer is yes. This is the study of epigenetics. The field of epigenetics is quickly growing and supports evidence that the environment and individual lifestyle can directly interact with the genome to influence epigenetic change. Epigenetics literally means "above" or "on top of" genetics. It refers to external modifications to DNA that turn genes "on" or "off." These modifications do not change the DNA sequence, but instead, they affect how cells "read" genes. Certain circumstances in life can cause genes to be silent or expressed over time. In other words, they can be turned off (becoming dormant) or turned on (becoming active).[v]

Many factors can eventually cause chemical modifications around the genes that will turn those genes on or off over time. These include the foods you eat, your home environment, and the people you interact with, along with sleep quality, exercise, and movement, or lack thereof. Also included in this list are living with chronic stress, drinking water quality, outside environmental toxins, and toxicity in products like home cleaning agents, skin care, etc.

The truth is we don't address our *negative lifestyle choices* until we get a major illness, such as cancer, heart disease, or an autoimmune disorder. The good news is that this means we can control our destiny and not become a victim of our genes.

This is what epigenetics is: making better choices in your diet, finding out what foods are making you ill due to food intolerance, taking more quality time to rest and self-nurture, and assessing your happiness level in work, home environment, relationships, etc. Become aware of your thoughts, and ask yourself if those negative thoughts and feelings are causing you stress. Our perception of life can cause a tremendous amount of internal conflict. A great book I would recommend on this subject is Dr. Bruce Lipton's *Biology of Belief*. Through the research of Dr. Lipton and other leading-edge scientists, stunning new discoveries continue to surface about the interaction between your mind and body and the processes by which cells receive information. It shows that genes and DNA do not control our biology, that instead DNA is controlled by signals from outside the cell, including the energetic messages emanating from our thoughts.

If you are interested in this process, I highly recommend reading this book. Dr. Lipton breaks it down into easily understood terms. When you start to bring that awareness to the forefront, the next time your body gives you a symptom, you'll arm yourself with the knowledge and understanding that you don't have to play the victim to your illness. It doesn't control you; you have control over your genes.

Now that we know about the importance of whole foods nutrition (how it lays down the foundation of our health) and how our negative lifestyle choices, our limiting thoughts and beliefs, and the lack of practicing self-care affects our cells, we can arm ourselves with that knowledge to shift our mindset toward taking back control of our health.

Make a conscious change from eating processed foods loaded with refined ingredients, toxic dyes, excess sugar, and zero nutritional value to a more whole foods approach (fruits, vegetables, healthy fats, whole grains, grass-fed beef, wild-caught fish, and hormone and antibiotic-free poultry.) Eat brightly colored fruits and vegetables instead of Skittles and other damaging, fake foods. You'll save money on prescribed medications, and the natural side effects will be more energy and weight loss, and you will feel youthful again. Your cells will thank you, and your life will dramatically improve.

In Michael Gregor, MD's book *How Not To Die*, he writes, "Whatever genes we may have inherited from our parents, what we eat can affect how those genes affect our health. The power is mainly in our hands and on our plate."

If you're interested in finding a Functional Medicine practitioner in your area, visit the Institute of Functional Medicine's website *https://www.ifm.org.*[vi] In addition, I have put together "Key Questions to Ask a Potential New Doctor" to assist you in your search. Some take insurance, while others do not, and you'll want to know what your investment will be before you commit. You can find them in the following section.

Finding the Right Healthcare Practitioner

The right healthcare practitioner can change your life. Finding the right practitioner may take you some time, however. I have had some amazing doctors and some not so much. You want a doctor who will listen to your issues and have open communication, while leaving their ego at the door. An ideal doctor, in my opinion, would have both conventional and functional backgrounds to see both sides of the equation. More and more conventional doctors are finding that they see the benefits of getting the training and education in Functional Medicine, as more science emerges.

Key Questions to Ask a Potential New Doctor:

- **How do you feel about nutrition and health? Do you believe that food is medicine?**
  This is an important component to treating you holistically. A healthy diet is fundamental to maintaining health.

- **Do you work with other clinicians—nutritionists, health coaches, etc.?**
  A nutritionist or health coach will help you follow through with the dietary changes the doctor recommends and work with you on lifestyle changes as well.

- **What will be your approach when treating my symptoms? What types of therapies do you use: i.e., dietary, chiropractic, acupuncture, or prescriptions?**
  We want to find a doctor who looks for the reasons why you are feeling discomfort and offers therapies to help alleviate them, as well as finding the root cause of your issue.

- **What types of diagnostic tests do you use? Does insurance cover them?**
  These tests can get costly, and you'll want to know the costs up front.

- **Would you be willing to take the time to discuss what my lab tests mean?**
  Understanding your lab work sets you up with a benchmark for future visits.

- **Will you be able to recommend vitamins and supplements to support my overall health and wellness goals?**

  Most Functional Medicine doctors will do this, and when you purchase supplements from a trusted source, you know you're getting good quality ones.

- **What is your opinion on chronic disease? Do you believe some can be reversible?**

  This is so important. A Functional Medicine practitioner looks at the whole body, not just parts to treat your symptoms. Their training includes how to find the triggers that are causing you discomfort, not just treat your symptoms.

- **Do you believe in the importance of gut health and how that plays a major role in our immune system?**

  Sixty percent of our immune system resides in our gut. Healing the gut is the first step toward healing your body, and understanding the foods and lifestyle factors needed will be most important. If a doctor doesn't agree with that, I would move on to someone who does.

- **Do you take insurance or cash only?**

  This is very important to know before you commit, as you will have many out-of-pocket expenses without insurance.

- **How much time would my initial visit take?**

  A Functional Medicine practitioner will spend one hour or more with a new patient. If you're not going to receive that time, it may not be a good match. Conventional doctors only spend an average of ten minutes, and that leaves out a lot of important information that the patient has not been able to share with their doctor.

- **What is the cost of my initial visit and follow-up visits?**
  This is an important question, so you'll know what
  your health investment will be and if you can afford it.
  You may be able to discuss financing, if needed.

Before you meet with your doctor, write down these and other questions you have ahead of time, so you'll be prepared. Your health is in your hands, and you need to be your own advocate. Do the same for your health and yourself that you would do for your children.

CHAPTER 5

Healthcare in the Modern World

Here are some alarming facts about the state of our healthcare:

1. **Cancer is the leading cause of death worldwide and the number two killer in the US, with heart disease and stroke leading the way.** Age is the biggest single risk factor for cancer. Consequently, it is important to lay down those early building blocks toward health that I pointed out in my introduction to this book. Risk increases significantly after age fifty, and half of all cancers occur at age sixty-six and above. According to the National Cancer Institute, one-quarter of new cancer diagnoses are in people aged sixty-five to seventy-four.[vii]

2. **According to the CDC, about 610,000 people die each year of a heart attack.** That's one in four deaths. Up to 80 percent of premature heart attacks and strokes are preventable with dietary and lifestyle changes.[viii]

3. **One in three adults are at risk for type 2 diabetes, but most don't even know it.** It occurs mainly in adults over the age of forty, although there has been a rise in children with type 2 diabetes rapidly growing each year, due to the increase of childhood obesity. A sedentary lifestyle, poor diet, and being overweight substantially contribute to type 2 diabetes.[ix]

4. **Autoimmune disorders.** There are more than eighty types of autoimmune diseases affecting more than 23.5 million Americans.[x] The healthy human body can resist foreign invaders such as viruses, bacteria, and parasites. The immune system is supposed to do its job. But unfortunately, things go wrong, and the body attacks itself. There are no obvious patterns in autoimmune disease, as it affects individuals at any age and gender, thereby making the process of pinpointing important genes extremely difficult. Yes, there's a genetic component in autoimmune disorders. We now have the study of epigenetics, whereby our genetic expression can be modified through diet and lifestyle. When you develop an autoimmune disorder, something in your environment, diet, or personal circumstances has to "turn on" the group of your genes that causes the autoimmune disorder. Through diet, healing your gut microbiome, and reducing the toxicity load in your body, you can redirect problematic genes, which will turn them off again, restore your immune system to health, and improve your condition.

5. **According to the CDC, more than one-third of the American population is obese.**[xi] Obesity-related conditions include heart disease, stroke, type 2 diabetes, and certain types of cancer, some of the leading causes of preventable death.

6. **One out of every four Americans takes a statin drug.** There are roughly 127 million Americans over age forty-five who take a statin.[xii] This is our conventional approach when treating symptoms, but it is an outdated model. Over time, these pharmaceuticals suppress your body's immune system, which is why you may be catching more colds, flus, and viruses, and you're unable to fight off infections. In addition, they also inhibit the production of coenzyme Q10, which

aids in optimal immune function and helps you maintain a healthy heart and blood pressure. Statin drugs offer you a higher risk of neurological diseases, from forgetfulness and confusion to memory loss. When you go to your doctor and tell them you have these symptoms, they will most likely prescribe another drug to combat those symptoms.

Many people are fearful of having high cholesterol. This subject has been the topic of a huge debate recently. Cholesterol is in all animal sources of food because animal cells contain it, just like human cells do. What Western doctors don't tell you is that decreasing sugar and processed carbohydrate intake is one of the best ways to control excess cholesterol. In Dr. Jack Wolfson's book *The Paleo Cardiologist*, he writes, "Tens of billions of dollars are wasted under the pretense that cholesterol is harmful. Handfuls of pills, side effects galore, and lost time for blood tests and prescription refills highlight the runaway drug train."

If we learn to change our diet and remove sugar, carbs, and processed foods, and eat plenty of fruits and vegetables along with healthy fat, fiber, and protein, we'll lower our cholesterol naturally without the need for drugs, many of which have unpleasant side effects.

A Note on Fatigue and Cholesterol

If you are suffering from chronic fatigue, cortisol could be the source. Cortisol comes from cholesterol. Cortisol is the body's main energy hormone and comes into play when you're under stress. Your body releases cortisol by the adrenal glands and responds to fear or stress as a part of the fight-or-flight response. Dr. Jack Wolfson also states:

"Cortisol production is markedly diminished in many people because of poor nutrition (sugar, excess caffeine, etc.), chemicals, lack of sleep, and chronic stress. By trying to decrease cholesterol, we are tying both hands behind the back of the adrenal gland and limiting the creation of cortisol."

Most Western medical physicians have little to no training in lifestyle modification strategies, such as whole foods nutrition, exercise, and physical activity, stress management, sleep, gut health, alternative treatment therapies, mind-body practices, and self-care. So, what do they have in their toolbox? Prescription drugs.

The pharmaceutical companies largely drive our health care system today, and they know their target market. These companies spend over five billion dollars a year on direct advertising to consumers. They relentlessly market the aging baby boomer generation, who are watching prime-time network shows. Now, when a patient walks into their doctor's office, they already know the name of the medication they want to treat their symptoms. The pharmaceutical companies sometimes market these drugs using cartoon characters, downplaying their serious health risks.

The average time a doctor gets to spend with a patient is ten minutes. If you read my last book, *Finding My Way*, you know that I went through a lot of inner turmoil early in life, and I was living with chronic stress. This chronic sympathetic stress-state caused me a tremendous amount of physical and emotional pain. So, when I went to my doctor, I was prescribed multiple medications to treat my symptoms. Those medications came with many side effects, including weight gain, brain fog, low energy, etc. It was usual for me to have severe mood swings, bouts of depression, fear, and anxiety, and insomnia. I now know that the reason for my suffering was that I was not addressing my negative emotions, living with chronic stress, dealing with a toxic work environment, and eating poorly. I lived with shame because of my situation; I always was afraid to speak up for myself, which led to feeling unworthy and having low self-esteem. And because I had a family history of mental illness, the doctors always prescribed me antidepressants such as Zoloft, Wellbutrin,

Paxil, Prozac, etc., as well as muscle relaxers to treat my physical pain. When I had bouts of severe anxiety, I always had my Xanax close by. Xanax is a tranquilizer that helps relieve short-term anxiety. I didn't know any better back then. I watched my mother do the same. She had her own pharmacy in her medicine cabinet. Sometimes, when I ran low, I would go to her for a quick fix, and she always obliged.

Years later, when I learned to address my negative emotions and the false assumptions I made about myself, I began to take holistic steps to treat my body, mind, and soul. When I did this, I freed myself from the prison of prescription drugs. Through my research, I learned why I was habitually in a toxic sympathetic state, much the same way I watched my mother respond to her life. She would go into a screaming fit, throwing objects—anything she could find in her wake—slamming doors and cabinets, causing her horrific pain for days afterward. Through my research, I've learned that during the first six years of a child's life, their subconscious minds act like computers, downloading everything they see and hear. This means they take in every situation and every response in their environment. That information is then stored deeply in their subconscious mind. It made total sense: why I was not able to handle any kind of stress, whether it was external or internal stress. I downloaded my mother's response to simple things most people take in stride, and as an adult, I reacted the same way she did, without even realizing it. My body remained in a chronic stress state. My muscles were taut and tense, always in a constant state of being on guard for the next perceived threat. I allowed only negative emotions to be worthy of my attention, adding to my stress and causing pain in my body and depression. To make matters worse, I would go to the doctor and was subscribed various SSRI medications, muscle relaxers, and sedatives to ease my pain. The modern medicine approach to treating symptoms is very backward. This approach is like putting a Band-Aid on cancer, hoping it heals. Covering up my internal conflicts only got worse, and I never got to the root of the problem.

Like a tree, if we don't nourish our roots, our foundation eventually weakens over time. We can't keep putting bandages on our symptoms and hope they get better.

I learned through my study of epigenetics that living this stress-filled way creates a chemical response in our bodies, altering our gene expression. When diagnosed with breast cancer, hormonal issues, and autoimmune deficiencies later in life, through my research, I saw that connection. Even though I also lived with food intolerances, after a lifetime of eating processed foods, my mindset, my perceptions, and my fears dictated my health. Without even realizing it, I was allowing my negative emotions to be the driver of my life, tearing away at my healthy cells, which altered my genetic code.

Living with chronic stress is one of the leading causes of epigenetic change. Long-term stress is the cause of numerous diseases, including cancer, autoimmune disorders, hormonal issues, digestive health, body pain, hypertension, insomnia, heart disease, etc. As we produce more stress hormones, we're creating an addiction to our negative emotions, and our response is the same. It shows up as aggression, fear, anxiety, frustration, competition, hopelessness, jealousy, etc. When we stay in this automatic pilot state, we prevent our body from healing and going back into homeostasis toward a more balanced, healthy state.

In Joe Dispenza's book, *You Are the Placebo,* he writes:

When we think our thoughts and feel our feelings, our bodies respond in a complex formula of biological shifts and alterations, and each experience pushes the buttons of real genetic changes within our cells. As long as you perceive your life through the lens of the past and react to the conditions with the same neutral pattern and from the same level of mind, you're headed toward a very specific, predetermined genetic destiny. What you believe about yourself, your thoughts, your perceptions, your experiences, your conditioned mind, is what is driving your future world.

Understanding this process will motivate you the same way it did me: to go to work on changing those limiting beliefs and perceptions and self-sabotaging habits, and in creating a new reality. This was the biggest gift I gave myself, and I want the same for you. When I purposefully changed my thoughts, my perceptions, and how I reacted to everyday life, using my conscious mind, I began to change the programming in my subconscious mind. As I did this, I rewrote my subconscious programming to reflect my new reality.

Understand that 95 percent of the time we are operating from our subconscious mind, while only 5 percent of the time, we are present, using our conscious mind. The conscious mind is much more powerful than the subconscious mind. The subconscious mind doesn't think; it acts as a recording device. It just plays back whatever you recorded. Think about driving to a friend's house. You're listening to an audiobook on the way over there; your conscious mind is aware of the present moment and listens to that book, while your subconscious mind is driving you to your destination. You pull up to your friend's house without even realizing how you got there. That's because your subconscious is running the show, without a second thought. That plays out constantly in your daily life. What we need to remember is that if our subconscious is not doing the things we desire, but rather is sabotaging those very things. We need to be aware of it and take action to change.

Your health and happiness depend on your ability to understand this and to go to work on rewriting your habits and behaviors. The goal is to create new circuits in your brain to reflect your new reality.

In the neuroscience world, it is said, "neurons that fire together, wire together," meaning that each time you repeat a thought or an action, you strengthen the connection between a set of brain cells or neurons. As the brain changes, the mind changes, and changes in your mind are a result of you deliberately and repeatedly changing your conscious thoughts to make a lasting change to the brain. So, if it's more joy, inner peace, and happiness you're after, you have the power to make it happen.

I was able to make lasting change in my mind, and you can change your mind too. I learned to reprogram my brain to reflect my conscious mind (what I truly desired—joy and happiness instead of pain and suffering.) As I did this, I stopped abusing myself through self-inflicted body pain (muscle tension), anxiety and depression (my perception of life), and feeling unworthy (my beliefs about myself.)

Today, people are more confused than ever about which direction to take in their health pursuit. There are many problems in our health-care system, despite the fact that it is supposed to be the best in the world at treating chronic disease. Yet, insurance companies will not reimburse for natural treatments, which can actually help people get off medication and reverse their symptoms, rather than just masking them.

A health issue is constantly challenging me, and still, I have fears of the unknown when a symptom arises. But I have experienced the power of being willing to bring a whole new awareness to my approach and my own health concerns. It's a paradigm shift away from everything conventional medicine has taught me, and it helps me rethink my approach when I'm not feeling well. Conventional medicine taught us to treat our *dis-ease* or illness. Functional Medicine is about figuring out why it's there in the first place.

A few years ago, I was having a hard time. I thought I was losing my mind. I couldn't remember names or why I was there when I walked into a room. My memory, focus, and energy completely vanished. I had a "wired but tired" feeling throughout my day, every day. I wasn't sleeping, which only compounded my symptoms. I would go the entire night and not sleep. When I went in for my annual physical, I sat in the doctor's office in tears, telling him my symptoms. He looked at me and said, "Do you think you could be coming down with early dementia?"

This diagnosis makes sense using the conventional medicine approach—confusion, memory issues, exhaustion, and a woman in her mid-fifties—early dementia! It was efficient—I'll give him that. But it doesn't address the fundamental problem, the underlying reason why my body was experiencing these symptoms.

More importantly, what would have happened if I'd agreed to seek treatment for that diagnosis? I would begin to suppress my symptoms with drugs and have to live with their side effects. This strategy would not help me address the underlying cause of the problem. I would become a "patient for life," wearing that label instead of reversing the disease and restoring health.

After that meeting, I met with a Functional Medicine doctor to get a second opinion. Because I was eating well, including organic produce, good quality meats, fish, and smoothies every day, I was perplexed as to why it was happening. I learned that even though I was eating healthily, my digestion system wasn't working properly. I was not producing enough acid in my stomach to digest my food. And because my digestion wasn't working properly, I wasn't getting the nutrients from my food. They were just released into my bloodstream and causing a host of problems. Then my digestive issues caused unbalanced hormones. Our bodies are always giving us feedback. A symptom is feedback that you're out of balance somewhere, so listen to your body.

Through Functional Medicine testing, I learned that my circadian rhythm was working backward. My cortisol (energy hormone) was highest at night and lowest in the morning when I needed the energy boost. At night, cortisol should gradually go down as our body prepares for sleep. Then we produce melatonin (sleep hormone) to help us sleep. As with my digestion issues, my hormones were not working properly, and they were the reason why I had been feeling wired but tired for so long. I was placed on various herbs, supplements, minerals, probiotics, and digestive enzymes to help with my digestion issues and bring my cortisol levels back to the normal range again. I worked on getting quality sleep. I needed to improve my sleep habits and get into a routine where my body would adjust. Also, I needed to be aware of anything that could cause me additional stress, as I needed to take good care of how I was treating my body, in addition to getting proper rest. Our bodies heal when we're in the parasympathetic (rest-and-restore) phase. When we're in the chronic stress (sympathetic) phase, we can't heal.

This whole process took me about a year. A long time? Maybe. But what is the alternative? I would have had to live with my symptoms for the rest of my life. In the scheme of things, a year is not a long time. And, as with everything I do, I learned a great deal about my health during this whole process. Now, in turn, I am teaching others.

Modern medicine has a lot of room for improvement, and with the alarming statistics of chronic disease on the rise, we can't ignore the importance of practicing preventative care. Don't let your symptoms rule your future. If you are open to looking at your health instead of looking at your *dis-ease*, you can heal!

CHAPTER 6

My Cancer Diagnosis

As I mentioned in the introduction of this book, I received my divine tap on the shoulder at forty-four years of age from a breast cancer diagnosis. I unknowingly contributed to my cancer diagnosis by the way I was living my life. I had a lifelong affair with eating processed foods and chronic stress brought on by my perception of my life and multiple medications to treat anxiety, depression, and full body pain.

My doctor told me that my cancer was most likely genetic, as my mother had breast cancer too. Her doctor diagnosed her with stage 4 breast cancer at fifty-six years old, and it soon metastasized throughout her body. She spent five grueling years with her cancer battle and then died at age sixty-one.

After witnessing my mother's suffering, I took a more proactive approach with a double mastectomy, followed by dose-dense chemotherapy. As I mentioned in my Introduction, it wasn't until after my treatments that I did genetic testing. Genetic testing helps you find out if genes that you inherit from your parents mutate, which changes how they normally function. BRAC1 and BRAC2 are responsible for suppressing tumor growth. When these genes mutate, it alters their normal function, which means you're more likely to grow tumors and develop cancer. My genetic testing came back negative.

It turned out that I didn't develop my cancer because of a gene that my mother passed on to me. My cancer diagnosis was due to lifestyle factors I wasn't even aware of at the time. Cancer woke me up to paying attention to the foods I was eating, my stress levels, and my lifestyle choices. My immune system was not great back then. I chronically caught colds, sinus infections, and viruses.

When we have a compromised immune system, we're more likely to develop cancer or other chronic illnesses. When we have a strong immune system, our body can identify and eliminate cancer cells. When we're feeding our body with nourishing, plant-based foods, like fruits and vegetables, those cancer cells can't grow. Every cell in our body has a predetermined life span. Some live longer than others do: for days, weeks, or even months. The cancer cell doesn't die. They live much too long and multiply. This process forms tumors, which start with a cancer stem cell. If our immune system is healthy, its design allows it to identify and fight off cancer cells. If our immune system is weak, overloaded, or suppressed, it can't keep up with the demands our body is placing on it, and tumors form. The good news is you can heal your body and starve cancer when you adopt proper dietary and lifestyle changes.

One great reference on this subject is *ChrisBeatCancer.com*. Chris's story is truly a remarkable in that, against all odds, he beat cancer through dietary and lifestyle changes. Chris was diagnosed with stage IIIC colon cancer in 2003. After surgery, he opted out of chemotherapy and used nutrition and natural therapies to heal. Chris is now vibrant, strong, and cancer-free. Today, he teaches others about the importance of addressing diet, lifestyle, stress, and the toxic burden we are placing on our bodies. Chris states, "Cancer didn't invade you from another planet. Your body created it. These are your cells. Cancer is you, your cells, your DNA. Your body created it, and your body can heal it."

Another great resource is a book by Dr. Kelly Turner, *Radical Remission*. I would recommend this book to everyone, as it empowers you to take full responsibility and ownership over your diet and lifestyle choices to maintain health. Dr. Turner addresses ways to heal yourself and your cancer and not to wait for that diagnosis before you pay attention to those things in your life that are not working for your body. In this book, she highlights nine key factors that radical remission patients used when treating their cancer diagnosis, which are:

- Radically changing your diet
- Taking control of your health
- Following your intuition
- Using herbs and supplements
- Releasing suppressed emotions
- Increasing positive emotions
- Embracing social support
- Deepening your spiritual connection

When I am doing my cancer talks, people are always surprised to know that a very small percentage of cancer is due to genetics (5–10 percent); the remaining 90-plus percent is due to diet, lifestyle, environment, and stress. As Dr. Mark Hyman stated in his *Broken Brain Docuseries*, "Your genes load the gun, but your environment pulls the trigger."

Your doctor is most likely not going to discuss diet, lifestyle, stress, and environment with you. Your doctor's job is to treat and eliminate cancer with conventional treatments, such as surgery, radiation, and chemotherapy. While these cutting-edge therapies can be lifesaving and important, they don't offer you a sense of control or empowerment. On the contrary, they leave you feeling like a victim, as if you have no control over the situation. This sets you up to believe there's nothing you can do to control your future. I'm here to tell you that is absolutely untrue! When I was going through my cancer diagnosis and conventional treatment plan, no one told me that if I changed my diet and lifestyle choices, I would dramatically improve my health post-cancer and prevent a reoccurrence. Instead, my doctor prescribed Tamoxifen, a cancer drug, for me to take and told me that it would give me a better chance of avoiding another cancer diagnosis.

At the time, I didn't know any better and did what I was told to do. I believed this "magic pill" was going to save me. But I had a lot of side effects being on that medication, including strange problems with my uterus (heavy bleeding, etc.). I learned that one of the side effects of Tamoxifen is uterine cancer. That's when I decided to commit to my own self-care. I stopped taking the medication. This was my personal choice. It is important to have a conversation with your oncologist before making changes to your current treatment plan. When I made this decision, I realized it was up to me to take better care of my body and be proactive about preventing a relapse or an additional occurrence elsewhere in my body. I began with a healthy diet, regular exercise, managing my stress levels, and taking more time to practice self-care.

When we realize we have the power within ourselves to live healthily, we don't have to become a victim of diagnosis or disease. When we consciously live through the eyes of prevention, we empower ourselves to know our choices matter.

Don't let the fear of cancer steal your joy. Instead, understand *the more you take care of your body, the more your body will take care of you.* Remember to embrace those simple things in life that disappear beneath our daily responsibilities: things like having a healthy social connection, spending time with loved ones, playing, enjoying quiet time, and practicing daily gratitude. We live in a fear-based society that causes chronic stress, and therefore, wreaks havoc on our immune system. Focus on those things that bring you joy, hope, and optimism, and eat a diet rich in colorful fruits and vegetables, and your body will thank you for it. Amen!

I shared my cancer story at an event at the Massachusetts State House, hosted in collaboration with the US Pain Foundation and the Hope Collective. As the moderator was reading my bio, I knew the audience would be taken aback by my words.

I began with, "I am grateful for my cancer. Cancer was a gift. Cancer woke me up to intentionally living my life on my terms. I would not be standing here in front of you today, to be of service to others who may be having a health issue, if it wasn't for my cancer."

Receiving a diagnosis of cancer can be a scary place, as we fear the unknown. Getting a diagnosis of cancer is the universe's way of helping you address how you are living (or not living) life. Are you living in fear instead of love? When I went through my cancer, that's when I began my healing process. I worked with healers whose therapies helped me process my own pain. Those therapies, along with chemotherapy, saved me. Going through a devastating diagnosis, such as cancer, forces you to go within and explore loving yourself again, the same way you did when you were a child. That love gets buried deeply inside, and we need to bring that love back to the surface again. There is always a deeper meaning behind a sudden illness. And everything you learn from your health challenge, you'll be able to use to help someone else going through that same challenge one day. There's your gift.

Sleep, Hormones, and Cancer

Healthy cortisol levels, your main energy hormone, support your immune system. Cortisol releases certain "natural killer cells" that help the body fight cancer. When our cortisol is not working, our immune system is not working, and we cannot fight off cancer cells. During sleep, the body produces hormones to help repair damaged cells, so when we don't get good quality sleep, our body has no defense mechanism.

One major study corroborated the importance of getting quality sleep when fighting cancer. A Japanese study of 24,000 women, ages forty to seventy-nine, found that women who slept less than six hours a night were more likely to develop breast cancer, compared to the women who slept longer.[xiii]

Sleep is a vital and often underutilized cancer-fighting tool, yet its importance is rarely, if ever, addressed at your annual physical. A lack of sleep can profoundly affect other things like brain fog, poor memory, weight loss resistance, mood, problem-solving abilities, immune function, sensitivity to pain, and low energy.

Not getting enough sleep wreaks havoc on your immune system. Not getting quality sleep (seven to nine) hours can make cancer aggressive and feed its growth, the same way sugar can. Our modern lives are full of sleep-disrupting stimuli, from electronics, hectic schedules, blue light, poor nutrition, late night snacking, and caffeine intake overload, all of which can contribute to poor quality sleep.

I find that truly the only way to address lack of sleep is to acknowledge that it is a very real problem and that it is causing you some, if not all, of the side effects listed above. Here are just a few suggestions to think about when trying to understand why you may not be getting enough sleep.

1. **Sugar overload in your diet.** Cancer cells light up when fed sugar! When you're eating a diet that is full of processed foods, sugary soft drinks, etc., your stress hormone, cortisol, is working overtime and may be throwing your circadian rhythm (sleep cycle) off balance. If you find that you have a chronic wired but tired feeling that is a good indication that your sleep and diet need to be addressed.

2. **Make sleep a nighttime ritual and go to bed the same time each night.** Understand how to wind down and how melatonin, your natural anticancer hormone, is produced by your body and is essential in regulating "sleep" and "wake" cycles. It is extremely effective in producing healthy immune cells and fighting off foreign invaders and cancer cells. A few ways to wind down could include a nighttime Epsom salt

bath, listening to soothing music, meditation, and breathing exercises.

3. **Remove electronics from your bedroom one hour before going to bed.** If you're lying in bed scrolling through your Facebook or Instagram feed, that phone emits blue light and has a negative effect on melatonin production.

4. **Dial in your diet.** Don't snack late at night. Eat your last meal at least three hours before going to bed. Watch your caffeine intake and added sugars and sweeteners.

5. **Don't exercise at bedtime.** Nighttime exercise interferes with your body's ability to fall asleep and produce melatonin. If you exercise in the late afternoon (four or five o'clock), you should be fine. Anything after that and you're more likely to have trouble falling and staying asleep.

Our body heals when we are in the rest-and-restore state. Paying attention to our body's signs and symptoms, especially when we don't get enough sleep, is so important. Once we understand the importance of sleep, we can begin to implement changes and set sleep as a priority as part of a healthy lifestyle.

You already know that a poor diet, unhealthy lifestyle, environmental toxins, and your fears feed into a cancer diagnosis. While there are many reasons for cancer, one of the *main* causes is unaddressed, deep-rooted wounds and negative emotions. As I discussed in Chapter 3, if we are living with negative emotions, including repressed anger, ongoing grief, anxiety, worry, and fear, these emotions are major contributing factors to our ill-health. I'm not talking about one disappointment or occurrence; I'm referring to *chronic emotional stress* that can increase your risk of cancer and its recurrence. Emotional stress increases a person's susceptibility to cancer by altering the genes that control the stress response. While toxic emotions don't necessarily change our genes, they do set off a surge of cellular changes that promote cancer.

Negative emotions, chronic stress, and the problematic foods that we eat, including excess sugar from sugary drinks, processed foods, pastry, pasta, flour, bread, etc. (cancer cells LOVE sugar) all play a role in feeding cancer. When we're mindful of taking care of the body and actively engaging in ways to reduce stress through yoga, meditation, quiet time, play, and social connection, and we assess what we need to change, our actions bring more balance back into our lives. This stress reduction, along with a good quality whole-foods diet, and the elimination of processed foods and sugary foods, prevents cancer cells from growing because there is nothing in your body to feed them.

When I was hit with my own cancer diagnosis at the age of forty-four, I was under a lot of stress and had stuffed my emotions deeply inside of me so that I could ignore them. After my cancer protocol, including a dose-dense form of chemotherapy, I was back at work full-time within a week of my last treatment. I returned to work with a vengeance. I wanted to prove that I could do it all, so I worked longer days, more than I did pre-cancer, and I disliked the job! But I wouldn't face my feelings and just plowed through, ignoring my emotional state. So, when I walked into my Naturopathic doctor's office, and he explored my lifestyle, my job, and how I was handling stress and my diet, he said to me, "Donna, if you stay in this state, you're heading right back into another cancer diagnosis." That's when I decided I needed to take my health into my own hands and be responsible for how I was going to live my life.

In the *HEAL* documentary, Kelly Turner, PhD, studied over 1,500 "radical remissions" from cancer and isolated nine factors common to all of them. The people she studied used over seventy-five interventions, but from her study, she learned that all of them were using nine interventions. *Only two on that list are physical.* The rest address the importance of our mental, emotional, and spiritual well-being. I bring this up because although conventional medicine does a great job addressing the biomedical aspects of our health, it doesn't look for the challenges of understanding the psychological, social, and cultural dimensions of illness and health. In Dr. Turner's research, she revealed the top social, spiritual, and emotional aspects that strongly influenced the patient's healing process.

Those interventions included:

- Taking control of your health
- Following your intuition
- Releasing suppressed emotions
- Increasing positive emotions
- Embracing social support
- Deepening your spiritual connection
- Having a strong reason for living

I talk about this issue a lot with my own cancer diagnosis. It wasn't until I addressed my negative emotions and those things that were not working in my life and learned how to stand up for myself by setting clear boundaries, etc., did I feel worthy of change. Through this experience, I realized that you have to come to a place where you do feel worthy. Healing is your birthright, so educate yourself holistically and bring back your balance. Through this experience, you will gain a sense of power as you realize you have to take back control of your life. We all need to address our negative emotions and get to the root of our issues.

The reason why your doctor doesn't address this information is that Western medicine doesn't recognize that emotional stress can contribute to the development of cancer, although Chinese medicine has recognized this truth since ancient times.

Getting healthy is not just a physical proposition. Until you truly address those areas in your life that cause your chronic stress and ill-health, you won't feel worthy of taking better care of your body and your health.

Stress comes in the following forms:

1. **Physical stress:** falls, accidents, traumas, and illnesses.

2. **Chemical stress:** viruses, hormone imbalances, blood sugar imbalance, or prescription drugs.

3. **Emotional stress:** family tragedies, divorces, financial issues, being in a job that you dislike, unhealthy relationships, not setting clear boundaries, etc.

If you are in a chronic sympathetic state, constantly running your fight-or-flight response, there is less energy and resources available inside of you to repair and heal yourself. Also, our systems become more acidic when in a state of stress, and this leads to inflammation.

Some de-stressing steps you can take are to practice deep breathing, which calms the mind when your heightened sympathetic nervous system takes over. This happens daily when sitting in traffic. You engage in that fight-or-flight response. Next time you are stuck in traffic, notice how you feel, and then take some deep belly breaths to relax your body. I use this practice a lot, especially when I'm in a long grocery store checkout line. I work on my deep breathing to calm my nervous system down. It helps!

Other helpful activities include exercise on a regular basis, a healthy diet, and mindful activities such as yoga, meditation, massage, Reiki, acupuncture, and play.

When we combine the latest medical breakthroughs with smart nutrition and positive lifestyle changes, we begin to reverse our symptoms, and in some cases, eliminate the need to stay on medications.

Cancer hits most people later in life, due to having a lifetime of stress, poor dietary habits, and exposure to environmental toxins*. Remember those building blocks I talked about in the introduction to this book? We laid those blocks down early in life. If you take action now, you won't be a statistic, and you won't be in the category of living with chronic disease as you grow older.

* For a full list of environmental toxins and things to avoid, see our Reference Guide at the back of the book under the section titled "Environmental Toxins".

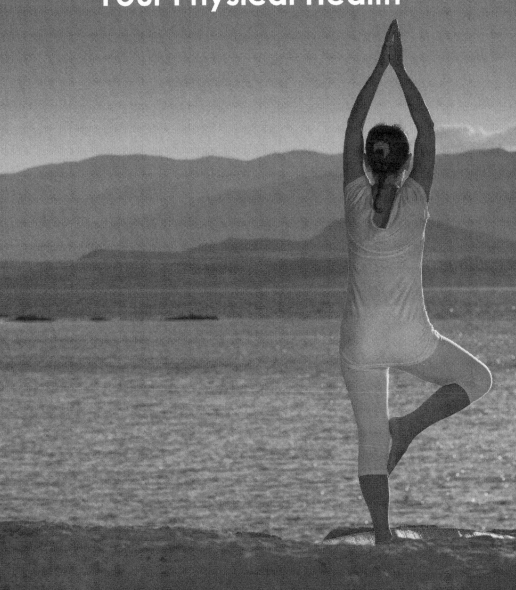

| SECTION 2 |

Your Physical Health

CHAPTER 7

Weight Loss Challenges

Why Most Diet's Fail

I want to tell you about the importance of knowing your *food intolerances* before you begin a weight loss program. Inflammation is a key offender that prohibits you from achieving your weight loss goals, and you can't heal inflammation if you don't know the root cause. I will explain step-by-step how to eliminate certain foods from your diet by using your food journal and doing an elimination diet, and then how to reintroduce them one by one to find the food culprits that may be prohibiting you from losing weight.

To take it a step further, I want to educate you about how inflammation triggers a host of other problems, including throwing our hormones out of whack. Especially during the menopausal years, when just one hormone is out of balance, it can throw off your entire system.

Living with food allergies, food sensitivities, or food intolerances can cause high cortisol levels. The most common offenders are wheat (and other gluten-containing products), dairy, corn, soy, sugar, artificial sugars, and processed foods. These are the foods that we tend to crave and overdo the most and are most commonly causing us negative reactions. I understand it is a total bummer to hear that the cookies and milk you look forward to for dessert every night are making you sick. But, in my own life, when I eliminated dairy, gluten, sugar, and processed foods, my health and mood improved. I am seeing great results with clients who follow this diet to uncover their own food intolerances as well. You'll feel energized, have mental clarity and an improved mood, and you'll lose weight. I lost a substantial amount of weight (twenty-five pounds total), and I had more energy than I did in my twenties and thirties. *And this was achieved without dieting!* The body can react with an immune or inflammatory response to just about any food, so the best way to assess what the body reacts to is with an elimination diet. I am including the elimination diet at the end of this section.

In addition, over exercising, extreme dieting, and eating disorders also raise cortisol. So, just like your nightly bowl of ice cream can affect your cortisol, on the flip side, starving the body of calories and nutrients can have detrimental effects on your blood sugar balance that triggers cortisol release and taxes the adrenal glands. In addition, the body can interpret too much intense exercise as stress. This is because the body can't tell the difference between running a marathon and running away from a pack of wolves.

When people have chronically high cortisol output for too long, their adrenal glands lessen the production output of cortisol. The adrenal glands simply can't keep up with the chronic levels of stress anymore. When you feel completely exhausted as soon as you wake from a night's sleep and it lasts throughout the day, you may be living with "chronic fatigue or adrenal fatigue."

The purpose of my sharing this information with you is to underline the importance of knowing your *food intolerances* and being mindful of how much stress you are living with, to not only reduce inflammation and lose weight but to keep your cortisol in check. In addition to stress reduction, it is important to be your own detective and use your food journal to uncover your *food intolerances*—to gain optimal health.

The following food list includes the most common culprits. I have included instructions on how to do an elimination diet to help you determine if you have an intolerance somewhere.

How to Do an Elimination Diet

If you're dealing with skin issues, poor moods, low energy, bad allergies, brain fog, or digestive issues like gas, bloating, or intermittent constipation, these are just some potential symptoms of food sensitivities. Food sensitivities don't show up as acutely as a food allergy. They cause slow-moving chronic inflammation that escalates over time. Chronic inflammation leads to disease, weight gain, and overall poor health.

Before you begin an elimination diet, start from your head and go to your toes, and make a list of everything you notice in your body, however subtle or long-standing the symptom has been. This sets you up to notice important changes when they happen.

Eliminate the usual suspects for twenty-one days.

Foods to Eliminate:
- Gluten
- Dairy
- Soy
- Corn
- Peanuts
- Hydrogenated oils
- Added sugars
- Processed food products
- Conventional meat and poultry
- Farm-raised fish
- Eggs (some people are sensitive without realizing it)
- Sometimes alcohol and caffeine (detox)

Foods to Include:
- Bone broth
- Probiotics and fermented foods
- Coconut products

- All colorful vegetables*
- Cruciferous greens
- High-quality protein, organic poultry, wild-caught fish, and grass-fed beef
- Healthy fats (olive oil, avocados, avocado oil, coconut oil, ghee, tree nuts, and seeds)
- Small amounts of fresh fruits

If you dealing with arthritis symptoms, try eliminating nightshades, including peppers, potatoes, eggplant, tomatoes, Goji berries, and paprika. Then add them back in to see if you're symptoms worsen or stay the same. Some people respond to nightshades negatively, and they can contribute to joint inflammation.

During this time, read all food labels to make sure that you're not taking in even trace amounts of these foods. You may want to keep a food journal during this time. A food journal is a valuable tool to keep track of your food intake, as well as your symptoms. You can download my food journal from here: (*https://bit.ly/2EF9B9J*).[xiv]

After twenty-one days, reintroduce one food group at a time. Incorporate it into each meal. After three days, assess how you feel in that timeframe. Notice any changes in symptoms between the elimination phase and the reintroduction phase. If symptoms do occur after reintroducing a suspicious food, you can confirm that this is an intolerance and eliminate it once again. The goal is to see if the symptoms clear up again once you remove the trigger. This process is a bit of trial and error, but it works. It should take a total of four to six weeks to accomplish from beginning to end.

How the Body Responds to Food

Weight loss seems to be a universal challenge as we get older. Some of us have had success following a specific diet and lost some weight, but what do you do when it's all over? Do you go back to eating all the things you ate before? For most of us, this is a familiar scenario. Whether you're following a compelling infomercial where they show real life before and after results or you've decided to try popular diets such as *Jenny Craig*® or *Nutrisystem*®, you're convinced this is the diet for you. Most likely, you know others who have followed this diet with success.

Let's look at the bigger picture. J.J. Virgin, the NY Times best-selling author of *The Virgin Diet*, says, "Our bodies are not like bank accounts in which calories come in and go out. Rather, our bodies are our chemistry labs in which complex processes take place that convert food to energy, the energy we store and waste."

Understand that when your new diet program convinces you that it's better to eat a less caloric meal, such as a sandwich consisting of processed white or wheat bread with deli meat turkey breast and a side of pretzels instead of potato chips, or even cheese pizza topped with vegetables, you're not fueling your body, you're depleting it. Also, if you are sensitive to dairy or gluten (most of us don't know this), you're feeding into your inflammation stew. These processed meals are not addressing your food sensitivities; they are only exacerbating them and causing inflammation, which will eventually cause disease.

What we need to realize is our bodies know how to use, break down, and digest a healthy meal, whereas with processed foods, you're in for problematic digestive issues that slow down your metabolism, all the while gaining fat storage. In today's busy lifestyle, we have access to so much processed, unnatural foods that we may be hurting ourselves more than we know. When looking at diets like *Jenny Craig* or *Nutrisystem*, these highly processed, prepackaged meals have limited nutrient value, yet are low in calories, so we assume we are eating right. You may lose weight because the portions are small; however, this comes at the cost of putting foreign substances into your body, which again causes digestion issues and inflammation. But this does not teach you how to sustain a healthy diet, long-term.

Also, when you follow a weight-loss diet, you will lose vitamins and minerals, your body's main fuel sources. When we deprive ourselves this way, it becomes evident. Symptoms will include fatigue, insomnia, mood swings, anxiety, and food cravings. It's no wonder we loathe dieting! Those food cravings will most likely be the things that prohibit you from losing weight in the first place. They are your body's familiar territory, and you will be looking for ways to get your fix.

Let's use sugar as an example. You eat sugar in most processed food products, pastries, cookies, ice cream, cereals, crackers, etc. You love it, then crave it because it has addictive properties that cause your blood sugar to spike, releasing dopamine (the feel-good hormone) in the brain, which creates an addiction. Then your body secretes a large amount of insulin—insulin is the hormone secreted by the pancreas that moves glucose (sugar) from your blood into your cells for energy and storage—to reduce your blood sugar levels. When this happens, it causes your blood sugar levels to fall rapidly. But because you have high insulin levels, it goes into immediate fat storage. When the blood sugar drops, your body craves more sugar and wants that high feeling to return, creating a vicious cycle. Low blood sugar levels create an increase in appetite, making you crave more sugar so you want to eat more, and the cycle continues.

Eating a high carbohydrate, low-fat diet creates excess glucose (sugar) in your body. When you're chronically eating many carbo-hydrates (in the form of bread, pasta, pastries, cookies, cake, etc.), then add on sugary drinks, flavored coffee, fruit juice, etc., it causes your insulin levels to rise 24-7. When insulin production is in chronic overdrive, the system stops working properly and the cells don't receive the sugar, so the sugar stays in the bloodstream. This causes insulin resistance. The signal is going out, but the cells are just ignoring it.

Think of it as a traffic jam. You're sitting on the expressway during the prime commuter time. You need to be in a meeting in ten minutes, yet you just sit in traffic; you can't get there. With insulin resistance, there's so much inflammation blocking the cells in your body that the important stuff can't get in. There's plenty of insulin, but nothing happens when it is released, leading to lots of both insulin AND sugar in the bloodstream.

When insulin resistance first starts, it's not so bad. Then eventually the cells begin to take up the glucose. This is why it often goes unnoticed in the early stages. But, as it gets worse, it becomes harder and harder for insulin to do its job.

When this happens, your body looks for sugar to burn instead of fat. When your levels drop, it craves another sugar fix. Then the hormone leptin (the hormone that tells your brain that you're full) becomes resistant as well. It is constantly looking for more food. When leptin resistance is chronic, you're unable to lose weight because you're constantly hungry. And if you're not doing any form of movement, exercise, etc., you're adding to that chronic state of storing fat.

A body with normal levels of blood sugar has an easy ebb and flow of blood sugar after a healthy meal. Your meal includes high-quality protein, healthy fat, fiber, complex carbohydrates, and whole grains. Your insulin does its job and raises a bit, but it doesn't have too much work to do, as your blood sugar levels drop off soon after your meal.

This is extremely useful information to know, as most of our weight gain is a result of food intolerances, manufactured and processed foods, excessive sugar, portion sizes, and not eating proper food combinations, e.g., healthy fats, protein, fiber, and whole grains in our diet.

When you stop chronic inflammation, you'll be able to lose weight. To counter chronic inflammation, we need to stop eating refined, processed, and manufactured foods, including anything made with white flour, added sugar, refined grains, rancid vegetable oils, etc.

Chronic inflammation messes up your metabolism and prohibits your fat-burning hormones from working properly. When your hormones are off-kilter, you'll crave all the foods you should avoid in the first place, from fried foods to salty snacks to sugary foods.

When looking at food labels, a rule of thumb is if you can't pronounce the ingredient, it is most likely an added chemical or dye added to aid in the texture, flavor, and color of the food product. Think Cheez-Its! Nothing is real! They make them entirely from manufactured, processed ingredients that mimic the taste of real cheese!

This is where whole foods nutrition starts. Choose fruits and vegetables instead of boxed foods. Fruits and vegetables are rich in flavonoids (they protect you against cancer and cardiovascular disease) and carotenoids (for eye and immune health) with both antioxidant and anti-inflammatory properties. Replace conventional meat, poultry, and eggs with grass-fed beef, hormone- and antibiotic-free turkey, chicken, and pork, and pasture-raised organic eggs. Eat nuts and seeds instead of chips and other highly processed snack foods. Choose organic produce whenever possible. At the back of the book, I have a quick Reference Guide all about foods to eat and foods to avoid. Conventional produce, hybridized with GMOs, is highly toxic and contains pesticides, etc. Why not give your body what it needs? Added chemicals from conventional produce will add to your inflammation because if your body doesn't know what that substance is, it will create an immune system response to fight off the foreign invader.

The Role of Sleep in Weight Loss

Other components to weight loss that most people ignore are sleep and exercise. We discussed sleep in the cancer chapter, as it is so important in preventing cancer but is also essential for weight loss. Sleep can make or break your ability to lose weight. Sleep will revitalize your immune system, balance your hormones, and rev up your metabolism so you can burn fat easily, increase your energy during the day, and improve brain function. So, the question remains—what is the ideal number of hours of sleep?

For most, it ranges between seven to nine hours a night. But with our busy schedules, we're averaging far less than that, closer to five to six hours a night. Researchers at the University of California-San Francisco have identified that only 3 percent of people can function optimally with six hours of sleep.[xv]

Not getting enough sleep will dramatically affect your ability to lose weight. Being sluggish, tired, and often irritable causes you to crave sugary foods, salty foods, and other processed or fried foods that are bad for you. These foods are not feeding your cells; they're depleting your cells.

Sleep deprivation raises cortisol, your body's stress hormone. So, if you are not getting enough sleep, you're always in that fight-or-flight response mode to things like heavy traffic, being late for work, etc. Sleep-deprived people have a weakened immune system and tend to catch more colds and viruses.

In addition, when you lose sleep, it causes you to want and crave more caffeine and sugar, which adds to the burden of not being able to get a good night's sleep. It helps in the short run, but then you crash and burn, and it becomes a vicious cycle.

Finally, not getting a good quality sleep increases your ghrelin hormone, which is the hunger hormone, causing you to overeat. Then, on the flip side, it decreases your leptin hormone, the feel-full hormone, the hormone that tells you that you have had enough to eat and prohibits you from reaching for that second serving.

You may be wondering what natural remedies can help aid us in getting a good night's sleep. First, you want to assess what you might be eating and doing throughout the day. How is your caffeine intake?

A cup or two in the morning should be ok, but if you're relying on it throughout the day, and especially later in the day or at night, that's going to disrupt your sleep. At night, try herbal tea instead. Or there is a product called CALM, a magnesium powder, which you can mix in a glass of water, hot or cold. Magnesium is an essential mineral that supports regular blood sugar levels, promotes normal blood pressure, and is required for producing and storing energy. Magnesium also aids in the relaxation process.

There are also some natural supplements such as melatonin, magnesium, valerian root, and 5HTP.

The bottom line is to make sleep your number one priority in your weight loss goals. It promotes a healthy lifestyle, as you gain the energy and endurance to tackle stress better, gain clarity on your "why" (your intention for wanting to lose weight), and take the necessary steps to understand what your body needs to find health.

Exercise More, and You'll Get Your Sexy Back!

You may be stuck in the belief that it's impossible to boost your metabolism in your fifties and sixties. But when you exercise along with eating a healthy diet, it is possible. I know you're reading this now and saying, "What?" We all hear that as we age, our metabolism decreases and our hormones plummet as well, slowing down our system. I address the effects of unbalanced hormones later in this chapter. A slower metabolism can cause weight gain, low energy, and a lack of focus and mood swings. This is the number one complaint postmenopausal women share with each other. While this is a valid complaint and very true, it can prohibit us from finding a better way, as we settle into that outdated belief. Aging = weight gain is a universal belief that has been handed down to both women and men for decades. If you visit your doctor and complain about your weight, you're most likely be met with, "It's menopause." (Or worse, "It's your age.") The missing link to this scenario is not investigating ways to help increase your metabolism as you age. Wouldn't you rather feel alive and sexy, have mental clarity, and get back the energy you once had? I'm not referring to going back to your twenties again, but most women, as they age, desire to look and feel sexy, regardless of age.

While there are various factors that contribute to increased weight gain over a long period of time, a decrease in metabolism is the main culprit. Even if your diet remains the same, you'll most likely gain a few pounds per year or more if you're not paying attention to your diet or eating problematic foods that cause chronic inflammation, such as gluten, dairy, soy, corn, sugar, flour, processed foods, and industrial seed oils.

Recently, I experienced some hormonal issues that caused my metabolism to slow down; therefore, I lost the energy I once had. Although I continued with a healthy diet, I noticed the pounds creeping back on. I realize now, more than ever, I needed to pay attention to not only my diet but also the time I was eating and anything extra I added back in that could be contributing. I am guilty of having a glass of wine or two at night to wind down. I also know that even though I have that healthy dinner, that wine (which turns to carbs and sugar) adds an overload to my daily caloric intake. When we are in our rest-and-restore state as we sleep, our metabolism burns fat. But if we're eating sugar and carbs at night, and maybe during the day as well, our body stays in sugar-burning mode, as opposed to fat-burning mode, and we're not able to lose those extra pounds.

I also realized that doing my regular Pilates and yoga classes, although very beneficial to my mind and body, was not enough to help me lose those excess pounds. I needed to mix things up and try a new regimen that would get things moving again.

Below is what I have found to be the most impactful and easiest to implement exercise and lifestyle additions. In a matter of two weeks, I lost two inches on my waist (and still losing), and I feel great. I am challenging myself every day and feel so much more empowered.

1. **Strength training.** Gaining muscle burns fat, a simple science we all know. You know how much I advocate for resistance training. Our bones need this, our body stays strong, and it guarantees you're going to boost your mood and your metabolism. And you'll look and feel amazing!

2. **High-intensity interval training (HIIT).** Cardio bursts (one of the quickest ways to rev up your metabolism and lose weight). When you start to incorporate HIIT training, you'll understand why it is so important to stay fit and healthy as you age. Nothing makes you feel less sexy than sitting on your butt all day and not moving. A sedentary lifestyle puts years on your age. It's a prescription to live a long, drawn out, unhealthy, and unhappy life. It is my hope that you don't go there! If you're unsure how to proceed doing HIIT, you can hire a personal trainer at the gym to assist you. In addition, there are more group classes, such as boot camp classes, popping up everywhere. One small boutique gym that I go to for my HIIT is Orange Theory. Their HIIT is a fifty-five-minute, high-intensity workout that gets my heart rate going and always improves my overall mood and energy throughout the day. Doing this workout helps me burn calories up to thirty-six hours post-workout. Now, that's mastering my metabolism!

3. **Start where you are.** If you are new to any form of exercise, it's time to figure out your starting point. Starting, no matter how small, is the key. Your starting point may be going for a half-mile walk at lunchtime, then increases as you incorporate this into your daily routine. Small steps lead to major improvements in your health.

4. **Intermittent fasting.** This is probably one of the most underutilized weight loss techniques. Keep a short window (eight to twelve hours a day) for your meals and snacks, and then fast as long as you can go. An example is that two to three days a week, my last meal will consist of protein, fat, complex carbs, and fiber and will end around six or seven o'clock. I won't have my next meal until noon the following day (a seventeen- to eighteen-hour fast). *Eating a healthy meal will move you into fat-burning, not sugar burning, so be careful to pay attention to what you are eating.* Some days I have a harder time with this, so I pull out my homemade bone broth and sip on that to keep me satisfied. I get the benefits of the collagen and gelatin, both antiaging powerhouses that help my body stay and feel young.

   Herbal tea works as well. When it comes to intermittent fasting, play around with this and fast as long as it feels right for you. You may want to go without dinner instead, and your twelve-hour food window would include breakfast, lunch, and a healthy snack. Then skip dinner. Use whatever works for your schedule and your body. If you suffer from low blood sugar levels, I would not recommend intermittent fasting. Always consult your doctor before trying if you feel unsure. When you're eating a healthy diet and eliminating those extra things that contribute to weight gain, you'll notice the pounds melt away faster using this method.

5. **Maintaining a healthy body mass index (BMI).** Maintaining a healthy weight is one of the most important things you can do for your health. A major focus of the Nurses' Health Study research involves evaluating how women may achieve overall healthy aging. Their findings were that BMI is an important factor in many aspects of

health and strongly influences the aging process. They examined womens' BMI at midlife and how it affects aging at seventy and older. Their results were astonishing. Women had shorter lifespans with an increased BMI at midlife of thirty or greater. It decreased their healthy survival by 80 percent, compared to those women with a BMI between 18.5 and 22.9.[xvi] This means that making well-informed, nutrient-rich choices is even more important as you enter midlife. To calculate your BMI, use this simple calculation: BMI = weight ÷ height in inches ÷ height in inches again × 703.

This is why it is so important to remember to eat healthily and exercise! You'll not only feel better, but you will live longer, and feel and look sexy and strong!

6. **Get your healthy seven to nine hours of sleep.** Here it is again! Don't underestimate sleep. It controls your sugar cravings, salt cravings, and your hormones. If we don't sleep, we are more apt to reach for that late-night bowl of ice cream to satisfy our mood, sabotaging all of our efforts.

The Role of Hormones

As we age and move through menopause, one universal complaint by many is increased weight gain or weight loss resistance. It's harder now than ever before to lose those stubborn pounds. What we often overlook as the main cause for weight loss resistance is hormonal imbalances. As women, we are extremely sensitive to stress and inflammation. When we don't listen to our body's symptoms, our inflammation only gets worse and can set off a cascade of unbalanced hormones. Some of these symptoms may look like moodiness, a lack of sleep, fatigue, a foggy brain, or feeling overwhelmed. These symptoms are signs that our hormones may be unbalanced and that it's time to address them through dietary and lifestyle changes. When we're in this chronic, low-grade inflammation state, "inflammaging" occurs.[xvii]

Inflammaging is a high-risk factor for age-related chronic illness and disease, where the hormones that help you burn fat (metabolism) cease to do their job and cause us to store fat. When your metabolism breaks down, no matter what you do, you can't lose weight. When your metabolism is broken, you need to look at the seven hormones that are responsible for the breakdown: insulin, estrogen, leptin, cortisol, thyroid, testosterone, and growth hormone. These hormones connect with each other and respond to the foods you consume every day. Let me use the most substantial of these hormones to demonstrate the importance a healthy diet, lifestyle, and reduced stress have on our weight and overall health.

If you struggle to get and stay lean during menopause, it's time to look at your hormones. You'll know because they continually give you signals such as food cravings, increased appetite, imbalanced gut bacteria, and food addictions, such as sugary and processed foods, the very foods you should be avoiding in the first place. And if you don't pay attention to the warning signs that your body is signaling you, such as weight gain, belly fat, low libido, fatigue, brain fog, etc., you're heading toward a chronic illness diagnosis.

The fat inside the abdomen around the organs is visceral fat and is the most metabolically active fat. The fat around the heart is similar. This is why so-called "central obesity," where the fat is around the organs, rather than the extremities, is the most dangerous, resulting in an increased risk of heart disease, diabetes, and stroke, as well as hormonal imbalances.

The main hormone that causes weight gain, inflammation, and chronic disease is excess insulin. When you're eating a poor quality diet loaded with processed carbohydrates, sugar, etc., your body remains in fat-storage mode instead of fat-burning mode. You already know that insulin is a hormone used to digest carbohydrates. Insulin's job is to move sugar out of the blood and into the body's cells to maintain blood sugar levels, ensuring that they are not too high or too low. Insulin resistance occurs when blood sugar levels are constantly high, usually due to eating a diet consisting of processed foods, sugar, white flour, gluten, and dairy, etc. The body's cells stop responding to insulin as effectively, the sugar is unable to enter the cells, and too much remains in the bloodstream. High levels of sugar in the blood place a demand on the pancreas to secrete more insulin. Over time, the pancreas is unable to meet that demand, and too much sugar builds up in the bloodstream, leading to prediabetes and diabetes. And because sugar is highly addictive, we crave more. Sugar is the reason why you complain about not fitting into your skinny jeans as you once did.

I mention insulin's role again because an important step to take on the journey when balancing your hormones is to balance your blood sugar. You can test your blood sugar at home using a glucose testing meter. This is a great way to discover what your fasting blood sugar actually is and whether you're keeping your blood sugar balanced after meals. Normal fasting blood sugar levels should be less than 100, although now Functional Medicine is saying eighty is the healthy range.

I've included a few test kits you can find on Amazon listed below:

- Bayer Contour Complete Testing Kit: includes meter, ten test strips, and ten lancets and/or

- Bayer Contour Testing Kit: includes meter, fifty test strips, and fifty lancets

The key to warding off this diagnosis is by paying attention to the foods you eat (see the table with foods to include and foods to avoid in the Reference Section at the end of the book.) You can balance out your blood sugar by avoiding problematic foods and introducing real, nutrient-dense foods filled with vitamins, minerals, phytonutrients, micronutrients, and macronutrients. Eliminate all the processed junk foods, vegetable oils, conventional meats, dairy, and gluten, and you're on your way to health.

Low Estrogen, Excess Estrogen, or Estrogen Dominance

It is vital for women to understand the importance of balancing hormones and their key role in weight loss as you age. Estrogen is a group of hormones produced in the ovaries that gives us female characteristics like breasts, hips, curves, etc. The most significant risk factor for having low estrogen is age. As women age and approach menopause, it is normal for estrogen levels to drop. Some women experience severe symptoms such as hot flashes, brain fog, fatigue, and insomnia. The conventional approach to menopause looks at it as having an estrogen deficiency, and when this happens, the doctors often suggest that you get hormone replacement therapy (HRT).[xviii] A study from *The New England Journal of Medicine* dated February 5, 2009, concluded that hormone therapy doubles the risk of breast cancer. Specifically, women past menopause who take high levels of both estrogen and progestin (such as in the form of Prempro) for five years or more have twice the risk of developing breast cancer. These same women stopped their combination hormone formula, and the number of breast cancer incidents dropped by about 28 percent within the first year.

While estrogen levels do decrease during menopause, many women suffer from the effects of estrogen dominance, which means they have too much estrogen relative to progesterone. Most of us are not aware that the foods we eat could be harming our estrogen levels. Have you ever heard the saying, "You are what you eat (ate)?" If you're digesting hormone-injected, superbug-infected, conventional meat, it damages your digestion, causing bloating, constipation, or both. It also raises your estrogen levels. Unfortunately, the significant changes in our conventional agriculture, whereby profit outweighs safe farming, has become the norm and is bringing on a host of health challenges. Women are at greater risk between the ages of thirty-five and fifty when the ovaries make less progesterone, which allows estrogen to dominate.

Another reason we have too much estrogen is associated with weight gain; you're dealing with a slow metabolism, and therefore, insulin resistance. Your cells can't absorb the extra blood glucose, so your liver converts it into fat. Then, starting around age forty, we become resistant to estrogen as our receptors slow down. So, our estrogen levels climb higher to receive those receptors. This is when we start experiencing more senior moments and mood swings, and we develop an unwanted "muffin top" on our waistline. Now we are in the full swing of menopause!

Traditional HRT Versus Bioidentical Hormones

Bioidentical hormones have become popular in recent years and are man-made hormones derived from plant estrogens that are chemically identical to those the human body produces. Estrogen, progesterone, and testosterone are most commonly used in treatment. Bioidentical hormones (BHRT) come in various forms, from creams to gels, pills to pellets. Bioidentical hormones are different from those used in traditional hormone replacement therapy (HRT) in that they're identical chemically to those our bodies produce naturally and are made from plant estrogens rather than synthetics. The hormones used in traditional HRT are made from the urine of pregnant horses and other synthetic hormones. If you are interested in learning more about BHRT, you can find a Functional Medicine doctor or Naturopathic doctor who specializes in hormone therapy in your area: *www.ifm.org*[xix] or *www.naturopathic.org*.[xx]

Regardless of your age, it is important to understand that too much estrogen, relative to progesterone, is going to offer you symptoms such as mood swings, bloating, insomnia, fibroids, anxiety, and depression.

Your hormones, including estrogen, are responsible for how you respond to certain foods and whether you burn off the foods you eat or store them as fat. If you want to find out your hormone levels, you can ask for a **female hormone panel** test from your doctor. This test panel measures the chemistry and hormone levels associated with aging women.

To balance out your estrogen levels, try avoiding conventional red meat whenever possible and stick to organic, pasture-raised chicken, turkey, eggs, lentils, or wild fish, such as salmon. These foods, along with high-cruciferous vegetables and a rainbow of fruits and vegetables can help reset your estrogen levels.

To read more on this subject, I would highly recommend *The Hormone Reset Diet* by Sarah Gottfried, MD.

Leptin Hormone Imbalance

Leptin is a hormone produced by your body's fat cells. Leptin regulates your appetite and how satiated you feel after a meal. It is also an adiponectin, which adjusts how you burn fat. When you are insulin-resistant, your leptin hormone stops working, and your ghrelin hormone takes over, which is the "hunger hormone." This may be the reason why you overindulge.

Chronic High Cortisol Levels

I've already addressed the role of cortisol earlier in this book but want to address the importance of cortisol's role in balancing hormones. Since cortisol is responsible for your blood sugar, blood pressure, and immune function, it can become a problem when elevated due to chronic sympathetic stress. It decreases your immune function, causes weight gain, and raises blood sugar levels.

Cortisol acts like an armed guard and is responsible for how you respond to stress. And if you're in a chronic stress state, due to a job you dislike, sitting in traffic every day, or a relationship that is causing you stress, cortisol can trigger a combination of signals from both hormones and nerves. These signals cause your adrenal glands to release hormones, including adrenaline and cortisol. Cortisol's job is to protect you from a potentially dangerous situation. But when it's in a chronic state, it can wreak havoc on your body's immune function and processes.

Thyroid: The Gland That Dictates Your Metabolism

The thyroid gland is a tiny butterfly-shaped gland centered in the back of your neck. But don't let its size fool you; it plays a major role in your metabolism. When your thyroid is working properly, you'll keep your energy levels up and your weight down.

The thyroid is essential to maintaining a smooth flow of hormone pathways. The thyroid gland produces hormones that regulate the body's metabolism, and having a thyroid imbalance affects metabolism, energy, weight, and mood. Weight gain may signal low levels of thyroid hormones: a condition called hypothyroidism. In contrast, if the thyroid produces more hormones than the body needs (hyperthyroidism), you may lose weight unexpectedly.

Thyroid problems can arise because of a number of factors, including stress, environmental toxins, genetics, nutritional deficiencies, autoimmune conditions, or other disease states.

Changes in thyroid hormone production can affect the entire body, from digestion to sleep to energy levels to weight gain. I would recommend seeing a Functional Medicine doctor or endocrinologist to determine if either one of these conditions is causing your symptoms and taking appropriate diagnostic testing to investigate further.

Another thyroid issue is Hashimoto's disease. Many midlife women are diagnosed with Hashimoto's disease, an autoimmune disorder in which your immune system creates antibodies that damage your thyroid gland. It is unfortunate that doctors don't know what causes your immune system to attack your thyroid gland.

The most common test that Western practitioners use to determine thyroid function is a stimulating thyroid hormone (TSH) test. If your TSH is elevated, that means you most likely have an underactive thyroid. The usual course of action is you're prescribed a synthetic thyroid medication to treat your symptoms. In some cases, when the test comes back normal, the doctor sends the patient on their way, even though they still have symptoms. Their weight remains the same; their energy levels continue to plummet. In addition to TSH, there are other tests that can provide a more in-depth look at this important gland. These include a full, comprehensive thyroid panel to include not just the TSH but also the free T4, free T3, reverse T3, thyroid peroxidase antibodies (TPOAb), thyroglobulin antibodies (TgAb), and more. Find a healthcare practitioner who specializes in thyroid conditions, which in Western medicine is an endocrinologist or, if you prefer, a Functional Medicine practitioner. These types of tests combined will give you specific information about your thyroid to get to the root of the issue. Their purpose is to point out if you are having trouble producing thyroid hormones, conversion, or attacking itself, etc. Many conventional doctors leave too many people undiagnosed, and when they are diagnosed, they're put on medication, which doesn't always address the root cause of the issue.

Some of the signs and symptoms of thyroid dysfunction include weight gain, hair loss (including eyebrow hair), chronic fatigue, a puffy face, mood swings, mental fog, anxiety, cold hands and feet, constipation, or dry skin, hair, and nails. These symptoms are typical of hypothyroidism, an underactive thyroid gland. This means that the thyroid gland can't make enough thyroid hormone to keep the body running normally.

Can a Glass of Wine or Two be Causing Menopausal Symptoms?

The onset of menopause is associated with uncomfortable symptoms, including hot flashes, night sweats, and insomnia. Many women reach for a glass of wine or two to relax after a hectic day, and as I mentioned earlier, so do I. What women often ask me is why do they feel the effects of alcohol more now than they ever did in the past?

The lack of hormones during menopause can affect how you metabolize alcohol. What you don't realize is that the very thing that you feel is offering you relief could be the reason why you're not sleeping through the night, suffer from severe night sweats, or both. Wine contains carbohydrates and can raise your blood sugar. Also, alcohol stimulates your appetite, which can cause you to overeat, raising your blood sugar once again.

As women (and men) age, they become more sensitive to the effects of alcohol on the body. This is because your cartilage and tendons lose water with age, causing your body to hold less water. The more water in your body, the better your body can dilute alcohol. We all should be drinking at least one-half of our body weight in ounces of water. Therefore, if you weigh 125 pounds, you should be drinking sixty-two ounces of water each day. In addition, if you have a glass of wine or two, you should accompany that with two glasses of water for each glass of wine to offset the diuretic effect wine has on the body.

Women absorb alcohol more quickly than men because they are usually smaller than men are. Women also have less of a certain enzyme (ADH) in their stomach than men. As a result, their bodies cannot handle alcohol as well.

A study conducted by Mount Sinai School of Medicine focused on the first-pass metabolism, which is when alcohol reaches the bloodstream.[xxi] It then goes through the stomach, where gastric alcohol dehydrogenase (ADH) isozymes break some of it down. They found that women have less of this ADH activity than men do, which means women have a lesser first-pass metabolism, and therefore, for a given dose of alcohol, their blood level is higher than it is for men. They also found that one of the enzyme's three components, glutathione-dependent formaldehyde dehydrogenase (x-ADH), is deficient in women, thus explaining their lower ADH activity levels.

The bottom line: If you drink wine and don't have any symptoms, at least drink a glass of water with it to stay hydrated. Try drinking organic wines with less sugar. They also have fewer effects from herbicides and pesticides. You can purchase sugar-free organic wines from Dry Farm Wines at *https://www.dryfarmwines.com*.[xxii]

However, if you're suffering from severe night sweats or insomnia, the best way to know if wine is the culprit is to eliminate wine for a week and see if your symptoms improve. You'll have your answer.

Healthy Fat and Weight Loss

Today's health headlines are filled with news about the ketogenic diet and how successful it is for weight loss and improved health. A ketogenic diet is a very low-carb/high-fat diet. It involves reducing your carb intake to a bare minimum and replacing it with fat. When you replace your carbs with fat, your body moves into a metabolic state called ketosis. When this happens, your body can be more efficient at burning fat for energy verses burning sugar and carbs for energy. A ketogenic diet can drastically reduce blood sugar and insulin levels. This can be a tricky diet to follow if you're new to keto, as the kinds of fat you consume make a difference. Fried foods are not the type of fats included in this diet. The fats recommended include cheese, avocado, meat, poultry, fish, coconut oil, olive oil, avocado oil, nuts, seeds, nut butters, eggs, Greek yogurt, butter, cream, bacon, olives, and the like. This is not an easy transition diet, so I would first have a conversation with your doctor before you attempt it. In addition, there are hundreds of websites, blogs, and books on this subject, if you want to learn more before you decide on this diet.

I remember when I was in my twenties and thirties, the latest fad diet was following a low-fat diet. I was not healthy back then, and I lived with chronic illness and a host of unpleasant symptoms, including fluctuating mood swings, gas and bloating, anxiety, and persistent weight gain, and I tended to catch colds, ear infections, and viruses more often. I didn't realize that my diet, which consisted of processed foods, dairy, gluten, refined carbohydrates, and sugar, was wreaking havoc on my health.

I was a proud subscriber to the "low-fat diet" craze, thinking I was doing well for my body. The media brainwashed us to believe that low-fat equates to being healthy and thin and that fat clogs your arteries, causing heart disease. Then the government and healthcare companies came on board and warned us to "cut out the fat." Looking back at the government's food pyramid, the bottom of the pyramid suggested six to eleven servings of carbohydrates a day, including pasta, bread, cereal, rice, etc. (mostly processed!) At the very top: one to two servings of oils and fats. The food industry jumped on board, creating all kinds of low-fat products, from low-fat yogurt to cheese, salad dressing, and crackers—creating the newest "low-fat is healthy" label. Do you remember the infamous Snack Wells?

Today, we're seeing the health benefits of eating healthy fats, not only for energy but also for the brain. That's because our brain consists of 60 percent fat. So, when we're feeding ourselves healthy fats, we're feeding our brain as well.

Unfortunately, today the average American consumes 150 pounds of sugar and flour in a year. Twenty percent of our daily calories come from sugary drinks, including sweetened soda, teas, sports drinks, coffees, and fruit juices. These liquid sugars are the most dangerous and the worst of sugars. They go right into fat production and storage. They are highly addictive, which increases our craving, so we want more sugar.

We now know refined carbohydrates are the cause of obesity and heart disease—not fat. Carbohydrates (those made from processed ingredients, not whole foods, like fruits and vegetables) turn on a metabolic switch, causing a spike in the hormone insulin. This leads to fat storage—especially dangerous belly fat. It is sugar and carbohydrates, not fat, that cause abnormal cholesterol and lead to type 2 diabetes.

Sugar is made of two molecules: glucose and fructose. Glucose is the body's primary source of energy. The body breaks down carbohydrates to glucose for energy (found in fruits and vegetables and unprocessed whole grains). Fructose can only metabolize in the liver, which turns into fat. One major culprit, high-fructose corn syrup (HFCS), is in many processed foods, including the low-fat versions. HFCS plummets directly to the liver, which then turns into fat. When this happens, we tend to overeat, as we crave more food because we are eating empty calories.

When we start to bring this awareness into our daily habits, we can begin to "crowd out" sugary, processed foods and soft drinks. Then we can begin to introduce nutrient-dense whole foods like fruits and vegetables, nuts and seeds, and healthy fats—olive oil, coconut oil, grass-fed butter, tree nuts and seeds, nut butters, and good quality animal protein and wild-caught fish. Below are some suggestions to help you on your way to health.

1. Work on reducing your high-sugar, caffeinated drinks.

2. Drink plenty of filtered water during the day. You can sweeten your water or add flavor using fresh lemons, basil, mint, or cucumbers.

3. Eat a rainbow of naturally sweet fruits and vegetables and crowd out processed, fake foods.

4. Avoid artificial sweeteners. These toxic chemicals mimic sugar and make us crave more sugar, causing obesity.

5. Exercise. As you begin to eat healthily, you'll have the energy to incorporate physical fitness into your day. Start where you are, and build upon that. The more you do, the better you will feel.

6. Make sleep a priority. Sleep is essential to your overall health and well-being. When we don't get good quality sleep, we don't have the awareness or energy to eat right, as we feel like crap and we tend to eat all the wrong foods.

Eating More of the Right Fats Will Help You Lose Weight

Below are some recommendations:

- Healthy fats: olive oil, avocados and avocado oil, coconut oil, and grass-fed butter, nuts, seeds, olives, and nut-butters

- Pasture-raised whole eggs

- Fatty fish and protein: wild salmon and grass-fed beef

- Organic whole-milk Greek yogurt, if you can tolerate dairy. (Full-fat milk has more protein, fat, and less sugar than the low-fat versions. You'll feel full longer because full fat protein takes longer to break down and fat makes you feel satisfied.)

- Flax and chia seeds: Both are good sources of plant-based omega-3 fatty acids, fiber, and minerals. Dietary fat speeds up metabolism and reduces hunger, which stimulates fat-burning. You'll eat less when incorporating healthy fats as you feel satiated after your meal. Healthy fat raises the good

HDL cholesterol. A ketogenic diet, high in fat, promotes more weight loss and inflammation reduction than diets low in carbohydrates and fat. In addition, dietary fat improves brain function. Remember—our brain is made of 60 percent fat!

Look out for the harmful oils—soy, canola, corn, sunflower, and safflower, as most contain GMOs. They create inflammation as they oxidize in your body and make cholesterol rancid. Instead, stick with olive oil, which is best on salads and not used for high heat cooking, coconut oil, avocado oil, and ghee (grass-fed clarified butter), which do not raise saturated fats in the blood.

It's important to note that it is carbohydrates, not fats, that turn into saturated fat in your blood—leading to heart disease. In addition, carbs (those highly processed foods, pasta, bread, muffins, pastry, etc.) turn on fat production in the liver, raising your bad LDL cholesterol.

Dr. Mark Hyman writes in his New York Time's best-selling book *Eat Fat, Get Thin*: "Sugar and refined carbohydrates, not fat, are responsible for the epidemic of obesity, type 2 diabetes, heart disease, and dementia." He refers to this epidemic as: "The United States of Diabesity." One in three kids is obese. By the year 2050, one in two people will become obese.

Dr. Hyman also writes:

Diabesity disease is due to carbohydrate intolerance. Just like gluten intolerance, many people are carbohydrate intolerant. For those people, carbs drive a hormonal and brain chemical chain reaction that makes it almost impossible to lose weight and get healthy. Diabesity affects one out two people in this country.

Now that you can arm yourself with this important information, I hope you can begin to understand the importance of knowing which foods are making you sick.

CHAPTER 8

Gut Health

"The microbiome is the next frontier in medicine. Understanding it and optimizing it is going to be critical to solving so many of our healthcare issues."
— Mark Hyman, MD, Cleveland Clinic Center
for Functional Medicine

D id you know that 60 percent of our immune system resides in the gut? Our modern lifestyle, diet, stress, overuse of antibiotics and prescription medications, and environmental toxins are compromising the gut microbes that are the basis of our immune system. Most people do not realize that inflammation starts in the gut. The gut has to deal with pathogens, as well as the food and drink you ingest to effectively ward off attacks and prevent illness. It is so important to have colonies of "good bacteria" in the gut. In fact, without the right balance of gut flora, your health will decline.

Leaky Gut Syndrome

When the integrity of the gut is compromised, it can lead to a "leaky gut." The body is no longer protected against "invaders" like undigested food, gluten, and bacteria that have passed through the "holes" in the gut lining. Bacteria and toxins enter the bloodstream through tight junctions in the gut that, when healthy, control what passes through the lining of the small intestine. When it doesn't work properly, it causes symptoms such as bloating, gas, cramps, fatigue, food sensitivities, joint pain, headaches, female hormone imbalances, sleeplessness, eczema, and psoriasis.

Scientists recently termed the gut your "second brain." This means your neurotransmitters (brain chemicals) are made in your gut, also referred to as the "gut-brain axis." The gut is the only organ besides the brain with its own nervous system. Your gut and brain are connected through millions of nerves, and the most important is the vagus nerve. The vagus nerve provides ongoing communication to the gut and brain and sends signals both ways. Think about a time when you got that "gut instinct" that something wasn't right. That "feeling" that reached your brain originated from your gut. They are intricately connected. What happens to one affects the other. Gut health is tied to every other system in your body, including organs and cells. This is why having a healthy gut is so important. The gut's purpose is to protect the body from foreign invaders to maintain a healthy balance. The gut works as a barricade to toxins and pathogens.

When your gut health is not working properly, even though you may be eating the most nutritious foods, your gut may not be able to break down and absorb the nutrients from your food. You need to create an environment where your healthy gut bacteria are working properly to take care of you and digest the foods you eat.

The causes of gut dysfunction go back to everything I talk about in this book regarding diet, lifestyle, stress, and environmental triggers. They include:

- Poor diet or the standard American diet (SAD)
- Environmental toxins
- Chronic stress
- Excessive drug use (including prescription drugs)
- Food intolerances

Your digestive system acts as the quarterback on the football team. Without a good one, the team falls apart. Your gut works with all the processes in the body and needs to be healthy to perform. Poor gut health leads to inflammation, which lays down the tracks for disease. Inflammation symptoms could manifest as chronic fatigue, chronic pain, constipation, indigestion, skin rashes, allergies, etc. Chronic inflammation damages healthy tissue in the body, leading to more illness and symptoms. Below are some suggestions and steps to take to begin a healing regimen for your gut.

1. **Chew your food.** The chewing process is the first step in good digestion. Chewing breaks down large particles into small particles of food and helps you absorb more nutrients. When you don't break down the large particles of food, the food is undigested and enters the stomach, then remains undigested when it enters your intestines. Then your bacteria will begin to break it down. This leads to gas, bloating, diarrhea, and constipation. Another sign is feeling exhausted after a meal. This means your digestion is working like mad to process all the big stuff. When you chew longer, you predigest your food and your saliva produces digestive enzymes that aid in breaking down your food, making digestion easier in your stomach and small intestines, and therefore, relieving those uncomfortable symptoms. The amount of times you need to chew your food varies on the size and texture. The trick is to take smaller bites to make the process easier, and you'll enjoy your food much more than when eating large chunks and wolfing it down.

2. **Know your food intolerances.** If you don't know your food sensitivities, eliminate the top trigger foods, including:

   - Gluten
   - Dairy
   - Corn
   - Soy
   - Sugar
   - Peanuts
   - Processed foods
   - Vegetable oils (like canola)

Some of these foods may be the ones that are causing you gut discomfort. Refer to "How to Do an Elimination Diet" (see page 83).

3. **Get the enemy out of the house.** Include anything with added sugar, processed flour, refined carbohydrates, processed foods, etc. Stop the use of all artificial sweeteners such as saccharin, Splenda, aspartame, etc. All of these foods negatively affect the health of your gut flora. Alternatives are stevia, honey, or maple syrup.

4. **Limit alcohol or eliminate during the healing process.** Alcohol is one of the main triggers of damaging the gut. During your healing process, limit or eliminate consumption to enhance your healing process.

5. **Introduce an array of fruits and vegetables.** Go for organic fruits and vegetables, when at all possible. Your healthy gut bacteria love these foods, and you're feeding them what they are supposed to eat.

6. **Be mindful of antibiotics use.** The purpose of antibiotics is to kill off bad bacteria, but what we don't realize is antibiotics also kill off good bacteria. They take out the entire platoon! Remember, our conventional meats are loaded with antibiotics. Therefore, we consume what they consume. This is why it is important to get organic meat and poultry and wild-caught fish whenever possible.

7. **Eat more healthy fats.** Healthy fats help heal inflammation. Include grass-fed ghee, olive oil, coconut oil, avocado oil, olives, nuts, seeds, and avocados. All of these are anti-inflammatory. And because nearly 60 percent of our brain is made of fat, your brain will love it too!

8. **Eat fermented foods.** Probiotic-rich foods like sauerkraut, kimchi, kefir, kombucha, miso, tempeh, and yogurt. Eating foods packed with probiotics and good bacteria will boost up your gut health.

9. **Eat prebiotic-rich foods.** These foods have the nutrients to feed your gut bacteria and help boost your immune function. Prebiotic foods include dandelion greens, leeks, walnuts, asparagus, Jerusalem artichokes, bananas, legumes, onions, and garlic.

10. **Take probiotics, fish oil, and L-glutamine.** When you combine these three supplements, you're promoting a healthy gut that allows for proper digestion by rebuilding the intestinal lining, reducing inflammation that leads to the restoration of good bacteria. Probiotics are living microorganisms that are living good bacteria. A probiotic supplement helps restore and repopulate the healthy bacteria in the gut. L-glutamine is the most plentiful amino acid in the body and supports intestinal health. Fish oil specifically targets inflammation, using the omega-3 fatty acids it provides.

11. **Drink bone broth.** The gelatin in bone broth can help repair the intestinal lining and reduce inflammation in our digestive organs.

12. **Drink warm water with lemon first thing in the morning.** When our digestive system is warm, it functions best. Adding lemon to your warm water keeps your body alkalinized and helps reduce inflammation. Warm lemon water helps keep things moving in your digestive system, picking up any debris left behind.

To investigate your gut health further, doctors who practice integrative or Functional Medicine can offer diagnostic stool testing in which they collect and analyze your fecal matter to look at the overall health of your gut microbiome. This testing helps diagnose certain conditions affecting the digestive tract. These conditions include infections from parasites, viruses, or bacteria, yeast overgrowth (candida albicans), and mold allergies, as well as poor nutrient absorption and low stomach acid.

Healing your gut is not always a clear path, and some things you try may not work immediately. The path toward health can be both challenging and confusing; it requires a lot of patience and diligence on your part. When you take steps to heal your digestive system, you'll feel much healthier and have improved mood and more energy, as well as a clearer mind, focus, and creativity. When you take the steps to heal your gut, the center of your body's health, your gut will take care of you.

CHAPTER 9

Health Benefits of Bone Broth

Whether you're sipping on a mug of bone broth or you add it to various dishes, such as soups, sautéed vegetables, or sauces, bone broth will provide you with the vast majority of health benefits, ranging from joint health to improvements with digestion, detoxification, reduced inflammation, and even skin appearance revitalization!

Bone broth is loaded with beneficial nutrients such as calcium, magnesium, sulfur, trace minerals, and more, as well as glucosamine and chondroitin sulfate, an important component in the fusion of connective tissue and joint mobility often found in pricey supplements that help reduce inflammation, arthritis, and joint pain. In addition, collagen in bone broth builds the cells in our brains and bones, and it rebuilds damaged cells in our intestines. And because of its liquid form, our body can easily absorb these nutrients.

For the Paleo lovers out there, bone broth was a way our ancestors made use of every part of an animal, by using bones and marrow, skin and feet, and tendons and ligaments and slowly simmering them in water over a period of days. This process causes the bones and ligaments to release healing compounds like collagen, proline, glycine, and glutamine.

Whether you're getting ready for surgery, recovering from an illness, dealing with pain and inflammation, or are looking to heal your digestion, bone broth is going to up your game when fighting your symptoms.

Let's peel back the powerhouse components of homemade bone broth for you to understand why this should be part of your daily health routine.

Joint Health

As we get older, our joints and bones become more brittle from years of wear and tear. And because bone broth contains tons of collagen, the protein that makes up bones, tendons, ligaments, and other flexible tissues, it's a natural alternative (instead of statins or vitamins) for taking care of our bones. The collagen in bone broth can aid our bone's strength and flexibility and gives our joints cushion and resilience. It acts like a soft cushion between bones, helping them glide more smoothly. Collagen also takes the pressure off aging joints while supporting healthy bone mineral density.

Improved Digestion

Sipping on bone broth is soothing to your digestive system because it is easy to digest. Also, there are large amounts of amino acids found in a bone broth that help maintain the integrity of the intestinal wall that, in turn, helps with the symptoms of leaky gut. The collagen found in bone broth helps improve digestion by ensuring that the stomach lining is healthy. Also, the gelatin in bone broth promotes probiotics, the healthy bacteria in your gut.

Youthful Skin Tone

Skin loses elasticity, and hair becomes dry with age. This is more prevalent when we follow a poor diet and are nutrient deficient. Sipping on bone broth is an inexpensive way to save money on expensive topical creams while feeding your body a nourishing, healing elixir!

Detoxification

Detoxification is key to healthy skin. We are living in a world full of environmental toxins, pesticides, artificial ingredients, and chemicals. While our bodies have the means to detoxify themselves, they often have a hard time keeping up with the overwhelming amount of chemicals we are exposed to on a daily basis. Bone broth is a powerful detoxification agent since it helps the digestive system to remove waste and stimulates the liver's ability to remove toxins. Bone broth contains glycine, which is one of the most important inflammation regulators. The liver uses glycine for detoxification.

Bone broth is so easy to make. In a matter of minutes, you're on your way to simmering delicious broth. I have used a slow cooker and Instant Pot. You start by boiling bones (beef, chicken, fish, etc.) in water with 1/4 cup of apple cider vinegar that pulls out the nutrients in the bones. You can add in optional spices, vegetables, and herbs. Broth can boil for as little as six hours or up to forty-eight. When using a slow cooker, I will simmer it for twenty-four hours (or about six hours in an Instant Pot on low pressure).

Various options when making bone broth include:

1. **Using one whole free-range chicken with neck and wings.**
   Eat a nice meal of roasted chicken; save the bones for broth.
   You can either freeze them for later use or throw them into
   a pot right away. Roasting the chicken adds flavor to the
   bones, which makes for a richer broth.

2. **Purchase an organic rotisserie chicken.** Use bones from
   that the same way; freeze or use right away.

3. **Visit your local farmer's market or butcher.** I have purchased
   organic bones there, including chicken feet. Chicken feet are
   not readily available at your grocery store and can be difficult
   to find, although some local butchers are catching on to the
   bone broth benefits and are carrying them. Chicken feet are
   going to give you a fine golden broth and will boost your
   broth's nutrients. Adding them to your bones will make a
   good stock very nourishing in glucosamine chondroitin,

collagen, and trace minerals. Also, chicken feet help make a beautiful, gelatinous broth. For people with allergies and leaky gut, adding chicken feet to your broth is the secret ingredient to healing, as the added collagen and gelatin in the broth not only helps the joints but the mucous membrane lining of the intestinal wall as well. So, don't throw those chicken feet out, use them!

4. **Beef broth bones.** I visit my local butcher to find grass-fed beef bone marrow. They are readily available at Whole Foods Market as well. Just follow the recipe found in the Recipes Section at the back of the book for the chicken broth and substitute meat bones.

Health Benefits of Collagen

Collagen is an abundant structural protein in all animals. It is a rich source of amino acids, which are the building blocks of proteins. Amino acids are responsible for some of the body's most essential functions, ranging from digesting food to building muscle, and it aids in the process of losing weight as well.

Collagen helps us build our bones, ligaments, tendons, and cartilage and supports healthy skin, hair, nails, joints, and digestion.

I have already discussed the importance of incorporating healthy protein into our diets. Protein provides the essential building blocks for maintaining health. Our digestive enzymes are made of protein, blood is made of protein, our immune health depends on protein, and our nervous system requires protein.

With the influx of smoothies, bone broth, and other high-protein meals, you will often see collagen included in the recipe. Collagen powders have become a popular option to get more protein without the added calories. I want to introduce you to the benefits of collagen protein and share with you how to include it in your diet.

Collagen and Joint Health

If you're living with arthritis joint pain, incorporating collagen into your diet will help. Studies have shown how people suffering from joint pain and joint swelling have benefited from the use of collagen in their diets.

Collagen and Gut Health

Did you know your gut lining is made from collagen? Collagen is in the gut's connective tissue and aides in strengthening the lining of your digestive tract. Amino acids, including proline and glycine (which are found in bone broth), also help heal and repair the muscles and tissues of the digestive tract. Studies have shown that collagen can help strengthen the intestinal barrier of the digestive tract.[xxiii]

Collagen for Skin, Nails, and Hair Health

Collagen is best known as an active ingredient in our antiaging products. Collagen helps us maintain the hydration, integrity, and firmness of our skin. So, when we consume collagen, we are contributing to a healthy skin tone, firmness, and youthful glow. One study revealed that taking collagen for eight weeks improved skin elasticity, especially in older women![xxvi]

As we grow older, we can experience weaker nails and hair loss. Collagen helps strengthen our nails and our hair. Hair loss can be due to genetics, extreme dieting, severe stress, or nutritional deficiencies, including a lack of amino acids. Collagen may be able to provide those important proteins for hair growth.

Food Sources of Collagen. One of my favorite food sources of collagen is bone broth. It's easy to digest and helps you reap the benefits faster. Collagen is also available in meat and fish. Make sure you choose good quality grass-fed meat, and wild fish, such as wild salmon.

What is collagen powder?

Sometimes we are unable to get enough collagen from diet alone. This is when adding collagen protein powder to your diet is beneficial. One of my favorite brands is Vital Proteins Collagen Peptides. My favorite flavor is dark chocolate blackberry. I will combine a scoopful of that with water and ice as a healthy snack during the day to keep me satiated. They also come unflavored and make it easy to add to your hot beverage, smoothie, and other foods listed below.

Most suppliers sell brands of hydrolyzed collagen peptides, meaning that they break down the amino acids in the collagen for easy digestion and absorption. It's so easy to enjoy collagen powder by adding it to your smoothies, hot beverages (tea or coffee), or baked goods to add extra protein into your day. I use mine in my morning cup of coffee. Collagen dissolves quickly, and it's tasteless. You won't even know it's there!

You can easily add to collagen to the following:

- Smoothies
- Soups, stews, and other one-pot meals
- Energy balls or bites
- Homemade granola bars
- Pancake batter
- Baked goods
- Applesauce
- Chia pudding or overnight oats
- Homemade almond milk or store-bought almond milk
- Egg dishes
- Dairy-free yogurt
- Dips and spreads, like hummus, guacamole, or salsa

You will find the recipe for one of my favorite smoothies, including collagen, in the Recipes Section at the back of the book.

| CHAPTER 10 |

Natural Ways to Treat Bone Loss and Osteoporosis

Another major concern of women everywhere is osteoporosis. I have been dealing with an osteoporosis diagnosis for over twelve years. Postmenopausal woman hear that the older we get, the worse our bones become, which sets us up for the chance of bone fractures or worse, broken bones. But we know that eating the right foods, eliminating damaging foods, and exercising on a regular basis, including weight bearing exercise, helps us to build a strong, protectant body while also building new bone. Exercise and movement, including yoga, Pilates, and strength training, can stop bone loss while building muscle and bones.

One past winter, I was out with my dog, Willy, on a blistering cold day. I made the executive decision to run back to our condo; it was crazily cold. Willy was happy running on his leash in front of me. Suddenly, he came to a screeching halt! I had no time to prepare. I went airborne over him and soon realized I was headed face-first into the pavement. I then crouched down and engaged my core, and broke my fall as both knees landed on the pavement first, followed by the crash of both hands. This scenario could have been a lot worse. Instead of landing face-first, my instinct told me to enable my core strength to break my fall. Even though I landed on both knees, and I was in excruciating pain afterward, I managed to walk away with only scrapes and bruises. Since I have osteoporosis, this scenario could have been a lot worse. This made me realize how grateful I was for my consistent yoga, Pilates, weight bearing, and HIIT training practice. That was the reason why I could get up and walk away without a fracture or broken bones.

In my first book, *Finding My Way*, I talk about a devastating response I had when placed on the medication Fosamax, prescribed for osteoporosis treatment. I was told that my chemotherapy treatments were the reason for my bone loss. What I wasn't prepared for was that medication caused a detrimental immune response in my body that nearly brought me to my knees. After taking Fosamax, my whole body was inflamed, and I experienced sudden, excruciating joint pain. Since then I was determined to treat my bones and my body holistically, without the use of drugs.

Osteoporosis happens when small holes or weakened areas are formed in the bone that can lead to fractures, pain, and a dowager's hump. It is more common in menopausal women over fifty. Often, you don't even know you have it until a fracture occurs.

There are many reasons for getting osteoporosis, but the ones I talk about below may be the most important because this is where we have total control. Arming yourself with this knowledge may help you eliminate the need to go on osteoporosis medication.

1. **Inactivity (a sedentary lifestyle).** If we don't build muscle, exercise, and move every day, our body breaks down, and we lose the flexibility, balance, and endurance we once had. That doesn't have to be the case, regardless of our age. Just ask a sixty or seventy-year-old who practices yoga. She trains her balance, core strength, and muscles to protect her when she needs them the most.

2. **Eating an acidic diet.** Acid-forming foods, including high amounts of conventional animal protein, processed foods, sugar, flour, and industrial seed oils (like canola), contribute to bone loss. It's important to note that when eating animal protein, stick with grass-fed beef, hormone- and antibiotic-

free chicken, turkey or pork, and wild-caught fish. Do *not* eat meat alone, as it is highly acidic. However, if you eat meat in a combination with an alkaline food, such as a fresh fruit or vegetable, you're pH will stay in a healthy balance.

3. **Low levels of vitamin D.** Vitamin D is found in cod liver oil, sardines, salmon, raw milk, raw cheese, eggs, mushrooms, and natural sunlight. Vitamin D foods help the absorption of calcium. So, it is critical to get this vitamin from your foods and, if not, take a vitamin D supplement, along with vitamin K to help with calcium absorption.

4. **Low Amounts of Omega-3s.** Omega-3 fish oil helps reduce inflammation. If you're not eating wild-caught fish like salmon, supplements ensure you're getting your omega-3s.

5. **Nutritional deficiencies (from a diet of processed foods, sugar, flour, etc.).** Add more whole foods into your diet that includes a rainbow of colors of vegetables and fruits, and crowd out the processed, sugary foods that have no nutritional value at all. Fruits and vegetables help restore alkalinity in the body.

6. **Alcohol, sugary drinks, caffeine, and high-sodium foods.** These foods may be hurting your bones. They leach calcium from your bones, yet another reason to make sure you are getting enough of the items listed above along with supplementation.

Natural Ways to Build Healthy Bones Include:

1. **Eat lots of vegetables.** They are the best source of vitamin C, which stimulates bone-forming cells. Eating plenty of vegetables also improves bone density, as you are getting plenty of minerals and calcium from your diet.

2. **Commit to regular weight bearing exercise.** Weight bearing exercise is probably the most powerful and impactful activity you can do for your bones. Weight bearing exercise (or resistance training) improves your bone density. One of the best ways you can control bone loss as you age is to add strength training to your workout plan. Also, the lean muscle mass that we all work so hard for decreases with age, so adding strength training to your routine will help you lose body fat, build lean muscle, and boost your metabolism. It's a win-win all around!

3. **Eat calcium-rich foods throughout the day.** The average RDI for calcium is 1,000 mg per day, and older women require 1,200 mg. But it's important to keep in mind that your body may not be able to absorb it very well. This means that spreading your calcium food intake throughout the day will work the best. Some calcium-rich foods include:

   - Raw milk
   - Seeds
   - Kale (cooked)
   - Sardines
   - Broccoli (cooked)
   - Watercress
   - Bok choy
   - Almonds
   - Cheese
   - Lentils
   - Yogurt or kefir

4. **Eat enough protein.** Eating enough protein is essential for healthy bones. Low protein intake decreases calcium absorption. Shoot for a minimum of 60–80 grams a day, and always pair with a good amount of vegetables to maintain a healthy pH.

5. **Drink bone broth.** Bone broth is loaded with beneficial nutrients such as calcium, magnesium, sulfur, trace minerals, and more, as well as glucosamine and chondroitin sulfate,

an important component in the fusion of connective tissue and joint mobility often found in pricey supplements that help reduce inflammation, arthritis, and joint pain. And because of its liquid form, our body can easily absorb these nutrients. As we get older, our joints and bones become more brittle from years of wear and tear. And because bone broth contains tons of collagen, the protein that makes up bones, tendons, ligaments, and other flexible tissues, it's a natural alternative instead of statins or vitamins in taking care of our bones. It acts like a soft cushion between bones, helping them glide more smoothly. Collagen also takes the pressure off aging joints, while supporting healthy bone mineral density.

6. **Maintain a healthy weight.** If you're in your twenties, thirties, and forties, you may feel the thinner you are, the healthier you feel. That just isn't the case for postmenopausal women. Being underweight increases the risk of osteopenia and osteoporosis. This is true for postmenopausal women who have lost the bone protective effects of estrogen. For postmenopausal women, low body weight contributes to reduced bone density and bone loss. That doesn't mean that being obese or severely overweight is good for your bones either. Maintaining a stable, normal, or slightly higher than normal weight is your best bet when it comes to protecting your bone health.

7. **Get plenty of vitamin D and K.** Vitamins D and K are both fat-soluble vitamins that play a central role in calcium metabolism. Vitamin D helps your body absorb calcium. Depending on where you live, you may be able to get enough vitamin D through sun exposure. Food sources include fatty fish, liver, and cheese. However, most people need to

supplement with up to 2,000 IU of vitamin D daily to maintain optimal levels. Vitamin K2 supports bone health by modifying osteocalcin, a protein involved in bone formation. This modification enables osteocalcin to bind to minerals in bones and helps prevent the loss of calcium from bones.

8. **Your plate should consist of 80 percent alkaline foods to 20 percent acidic foods.** Animal protein is highly acidic when consumed on its own and can leach calcium from your bones. When consuming animal protein, it is important to include a healthy amount of alkaline foods along with it. Only consume animal protein from animals that lived in their natural habitat. High quality, grass-fed beef and antibiotic- and hormone-free poultry, eggs, pork, and wild-caught seafood are best for you.

To keep your proper balance while eating the proteins listed above, be sure to include deeply colored vegetables and fresh fruit to keep your pH balanced.

Below is a list of *acidifying foods*. Always combine with alkalizing foods to restore your body's pH:

- Meat, poultry, fish, and seafood
- Eggs
- Cheese
- Animal fats, such as lard
- Vegetable oils, margarine, and refined oils*
- Whole grains, wheat, oats, and millet
- Bread, pasta, cereal flakes, and other grain-based foods*
- Sweets, pastries, and syrups*
- Walnuts, hazelnuts, and pumpkin seeds

- Legumes (beans and peas, except lentils, which are alkaline-forming)
- Commercially manufactured sweet drinks, sodas*
- Coffee, tea, cocoa, and wine
- Condiments—mayonnaise, mustard, and ketchup
- Medications (acid reflux meds and corticosteroids)
- Alcohol use
- Caffeine
- Cigarette smoking*

*Avoid these, as they can cause inflammation.

Below is a list of *alkalinizing* foods:

- Potatoes, including sweet potatoes
- All deep green vegetables, raw or cooked: salad greens, green beans, cabbage, Brussel sprouts, kale, cauliflower, celery, squash, etc.
- Deep-colored vegetables: carrots, beets, and peppers (except tomatoes, for some people)
- Herbs and spices
- Bananas
- Almonds, brazil nuts, and chestnuts
- Alkaline mineral waters
- Almond milk and coconut milk
- Avocados
- Cold-pressed oils (avocado, olive, flax, or coconut)
- Cold-pressed juices
- Sprouted bread
- Herbal teas
- Lentils, lima beans, soy beans, and white beans
- Amaranth, buckwheat, chia/salba, kamut, millet, and quinoa

9. **Include foods high in magnesium and zinc.** Magnesium and zinc are two very important minerals for bone health. Magnesium helps to convert vitamin D into the active form that promotes calcium absorption.

Foods that are rich in magnesium include:

- Dark chocolate
- Avocados
- Nuts (almonds, cashews, and Brazil nuts)
- Legumes
- Seeds (including flax, pumpkin, and chia seeds; pumpkin seeds are a particularly good source, with 150 mg in a 1-oz. serving!)
- Bananas
- Leafy greens (kale, spinach, collard greens, turnip greens, and mustard greens)
- Fatty fish (salmon, mackerel, and halibut)
- Whole grains (wheat, oats and barley, buckwheat, and quinoa)

Zinc is a trace mineral needed in very small amounts. Zinc promotes the formation of bone-building cells and prevents the excessive breakdown of bone. Good sources of zinc include beef, shrimp, spinach, flaxseeds, oysters, and pumpkin seeds.

10. **Consume foods high in omega-3 fats.** Omega-3 fatty acids are well known for their anti-inflammatory effects and have been found to promote the formation of new bone and protect against bone loss in older adults. Omega-3 fats can be found in fatty fish, chia seeds, flaxseeds, and walnuts.

In summary, eating a diet containing 80 percent alkalinizing foods to 20 percent acidic foods will restore and maintain your body's healthy pH balance, as well as reducing inflammation and improving your overall health. Consider taking calcium, vitamin D, vitamin K2, and omega-3 fish oil, as well as magnesium supplements to compliment your bone health, if you feel you're not getting enough from your diet. And remember to include weight bearing exercise to promote a strong body and strong bones.

Your body is capable of building and strengthening bone on its own. If you're concerned about your risks of excessive bone loss, these natural nutritional and lifestyle changes can be powerful protectors of your bones, as well as your health.

CHAPTER 11

Eating Paleo for Health and Weight Loss

As a holistic health coach, I have studied numerous dietary theories, and I have come to realize all of the conflicting information out there is confusing to most people. How do we know if a certain diet is the right one?

There is no one-size-fits-all approach to nutrition. However, when we take appropriate steps to eliminate and "crowd out" processed foods, like highly refined white flour products, sugar, gluten, and dairy, we see significant improvements in our health.

In my own life, when I took steps to eliminate gluten, dairy, and sugar from my diet, I was able to reverse a diagnosed autoimmune disease. I had support and guidance through a Naturopath. I learned that I needed to change my perspective on food and to realize that food is medicine. I shifted my awareness around healthy eating and asked myself whether my food choice was going to give me health and energy or if it was going to deplete my health and drain my energy? I was in a place where I had to decide to clean up my diet or live with chronic pain and exhaustion. When I eliminated the foods that caused inflammation in my body and introduced nutrient-dense whole foods, organic fruits and vegetables, grass-fed beef, antibiotic-free chicken and turkey, and wild-caught fish, I found my health.

I also eliminated grains and legumes from my diet because they were contributing to my inflammation. When I began to see my joint pain improve, my energy come back, my brain fog lift, and improvements in my sleep, I was hooked. That's when I researched my diet further and found information on the Paleo lifestyle diet. Paleo is not about eating high or low carbs, as many believe. Rather, its foundation is all about food quality: the highly satiating nature of unprocessed foods.

I prefer to call it "Paleo lifestyle" and not a diet. The word "diet" seems too restrictive. In my Paleo lifestyle, I am fully satisfied, and I don't feel deprived. The more nutrient-dense foods I eat, the more I want. I no longer have the desire to reach for that Cheez-It box to get my fix.

Looking back, I was living with an addiction to processed foods, without even realizing it. *Do you ever wonder why you can't eat just one Doritos chip?* The food industry knows how to manipulate processed food products, encouraging the consumer to crave more of a bad thing. When I cleaned up my diet, the natural benefit was weight loss: twenty-five pounds in total, and I have kept it off. I no longer feel the need to count calories the way I did in the past.

Research shows that a Paleo lifestyle is more satiating per calorie than either a Mediterranean diet or a low-fat diet. That means it's more filling for the same number of calories, compared to other popular diet methods. This is crucial for weight loss since it helps you eat less without fighting hunger or counting calories.

Here are some basic rules of Paleo:

1. **Remove wheat, sugar, grains, legumes, and dairy, as well as all processed, fake foods and sugary products.** Also remove refined vegetable oils and replace them with healthy fats:

   - Ghee (clarified butter)
   - Coconut oil
   - Extra-virgin olive oil
   - Macadamia nut oil
   - Avocado oil
   - Toasted sesame oil
   - Rendered bacon fat (pasture-raised, organic)

2. **Use in place of white flours and starches:**
   - Almond flour
   - Coconut flour
   - Arrowroot flour
   - Tapioca flour
   - Baking soda
   - Psyllium husk
   - Cream of tartar

3. **Replace conventional meats, chicken, turkey, pork, and eggs with organic, pasture-raised, grass-fed meat, and eggs.**

4. **Begin an exercise program.** Move, walk, run, swim, or do yoga, Pilates, resistance training, etc.

5. **Replace milk, cream, and yogurt with whipped cashews, coconut, or almond milk.**

6. **Replace rice and potatoes with cauliflower* or celery root.** (See recipe for mashed cauliflower and cauliflower rice in Recipe Section at the back of this book.)

7. **Replace soy sauce with coconut aminos and fish sauce.**

A Healthy Snapshot of What to Eat on Paleo

- Grass-fed meats
- Pasture-raised chicken, turkey, and pork free of hormones and antibiotics
- Wild-caught fish and seafood
- Organic vegetables
- Organic fruits (for weight loss, limit to berries)
- Nuts and seeds (raw and organic; for weight loss, limit to one-fourth cup daily)
- Healthy fats and oils (see list on page 132)

1. **Sustainable seafood.** Wild or wild-caught fish indicates that the fish was spawned, lived in, and was caught in the wild in their natural habitat. This is the ideal circumstance. When buying fish, you can find very helpful seafood guides on the Environmental Defense Fund website:
   http://seafood.edf.org/guide/best/healthy.[xxv]
   In addition, the Monterey Bay Aquarium maintains a free list of the most sustainable seafood choices.
   Visit *https://www.MontereyBayAquarium.com* for more information.

2. **Sustainable meats:** Visit *https://www.GrassLandBeef.com.*[xxvi] US Wellness Meats is an online company that sells sustainably farmed meat products. In addition, more and more grocery stores are stocking local farm meat products. Look for labels that say "grass-fed," meaning the animals ate grass, their natural diet, rather than grains. In addition to being more humane, grass-fed meat is more lean and lower in fat and calories than grain-fed meat. Grass-fed animals are not fed grain or animal by-products, synthetic hormones, or antibiotics to promote growth or prevent disease.

3. **Pasture-raised chicken, turkey, and pork (antibiotic- and hormone-free).** Antibiotic-free means that the rancher did not feed the animal antibiotics during its lifetime. Other phrases may say: "no antibiotics administered" or "raised without antibiotics." The US Department of Agriculture (USDA) doesn't allow farmers to feed hormones to poultry or pork—so there's no reason to choose products labeled "hormone-free."

Another diet similar to Paleo is Whole 30. I like this diet because (just like Paleo) it removes all processed and conventional meats and food products that have added sugar, refined flours, gluten, dairy, corn, soy, and vegetable oils and takes it down to clean eating with high-quality protein and organic, non-GMO vegetables, fruit, complex carbohydrates, and fiber.

The success rate of people who try the Whole 30 approach is high because this diet insists you eliminate all the bad stuff stated above for thirty days. After thirty days, you reintroduce each ingredient back in, one at a time, and notice how your body feels. This approach is very similar to an elimination diet. When I present this information in my workshops, I talk about eliminating foods that may be causing you inflammation. It is the first step in figuring out why you're not losing weight. The usual food culprits that cause inflammation in the body are soy, corn, dairy, gluten, peanuts, sugar, artificial sweeteners, and processed foods. These ingredients are in most processed foods and vary depending on the food product. In addition, they are made with genetically modified organisms (GMOs), which is another reason to avoid them.

Once you do the Whole 30 diet for thirty days, then reintroduce foods like dairy back in, you may find that you're fine with it. In that case, proceed. You may find that gluten-containing products are causing you symptoms like joint pain, digestive issues, and brain fog. That's a clear example of a food intolerance, and you need to avoid it altogether. Last, when you introduce processed foods back in, you will not want them, either because you're feeling so good or because they don't taste the same as they did before your health journey. They also lack vitamins and nutrients, which is why you're aiming to eat more whole foods. For me, when I gave up Cheez-Its, I thought I would miss them. But after several years, I was curious about how they would taste. So I gave it a try. That delicious cheese flavor was gone! It was like chewing on a piece of cardboard with a pathetic, cheese-like flavor. You'll notice that your taste buds will change as you introduce real, healthy foods into your diet. That's worth your time and investments, not to mention the money you save subscribing to diet plans that don't work!

I hope you give yourself this gift of health and you understand the difference between dieting and whole foods nutrition. Once you understand this concept, you'll equip yourself with the knowledge to know better when the next fad diet comes along, and you will be ready to greet your new life with gusto!

Helpful Tools for Cooking Paleo

1. **Buy a spiralizer.** It will be your best friend. Although many supermarkets sell prepackaged spiralized zucchini and summer squash, conventional zucchini and summer squash could contain GMOs. A spiralizer can help with so many vegetables, you will wonder why you waited so long to own one.

2. **If you don't already have one, purchase a Crock-Pot.** It will make your busy life that much easier. Throw all your ingredients into the pot in the morning, and then come home to a full meal with plenty of leftovers for the week.

3. **Purchase a Vitamix.** They are expensive, but a Vitamix is hands down one of the best ways to incorporate more nutrient-dense fruits and vegetables into your daily diet. I use mine every day and couldn't live without my morning smoothies. A Vitamix investment can range anywhere from $400–$750, depending on the model. I have two: one at my lake house and one at home, and I use them daily for smoothies and soups. I have been using my Vitamix for over four years, and it still works great. The health benefits alone make this a winner!

Portion Size Guidelines

There can be a lot of confusion around proteins and fats portion sizes when eating Paleo. Portion sizes vary depending on the size of the person, activity level, and overall caloric needs. As a five-foot-two female, I stay on the lower end of the chart for protein, fats, non-starchy vegetables, and fruit. I have unlimited amounts of non-starchy vegetables; that's when I add a mixed green salad or double up on my vegetables in lieu of non-starchy vegetables. I feel fully satisfied eating this way. You can play around with your body weight and height to find what works for you. The chart below is a quick reference. The portion recommendations may be increased or decreased, depending on your specific needs.

Protein	Woman: 3–8 oz. (meals) Men: 8–10 oz. (meals)
Non-Starchy Vegetables	Unlimited, unless it is drowning in fats and oils. Limit to 1/2–1 c.
Starchy Vegetables	Women: 1/2–1 c. with meals Men: 1 and 1/2 c. with meals
Snacks, nuts and seeds	Woman: 2–4 oz. Men: 3–6 oz.
Fruits	Cut larger fruits in half or smaller Depends on your caloric goal
Fats and Oils*	Women: 1–2 Tbsp. Men: 2–4 Tbsp.

*When cooking with oil, a rule of thumb is to use two tablespoons. In addition, when you add healthy fats to your meals, you'll feel more satiated without the need to eat more food. Remember, Paleo is a lifestyle, not a diet. If you just eat real food, you'll find your health!

CHAPTER 12

Smoothies

My mission as a health coach and author is to teach you ways to eliminate the foods that cause inflammation and ill-health. One of the quickest ways to do this is with smoothies. Fresh smoothies have a variety of vitamins, minerals, amino acids, and healthy fats, and lots of fiber! In addition, making smoothies is the easiest way to incorporate more leafy greens into your diet.

Smoothies also aid in our body's hydration. Most of us are not drinking enough water. Instead, we're drinking sugary soft drinks, flavored coffees, teas, and fruit juices. As a result, we are seriously dehydrated and nutrient deficient, which leads to food cravings. And, unfortunately, the foods we crave are the foods that cause us harm, not healthy foods that are good for us.

There are many benefits to adding dark leafy greens to your day, and some of those benefits include aiding your body's detoxification process, glowing skin, increased energy, fighting free radicals with high levels of antioxidants, and improved bone health.

The Basic Building Blocks of a Green Smoothie

1. **Dark, leafy green vegetables** like kale, spinach, lettuce, Swiss chard, and mustard, collard, and dandelion greens provide you with health-sustaining doses of folate, potassium, calcium, fiber, and vitamins A, C, and K.

2. **Fruits**, such as strawberries, blueberries, blackberries, raspberries, lemons, limes, bananas, dates, and green apples are natural sources of vitamins and minerals and dietary fiber.

3. **Hydration fruits and vegetables,** including celery, cucumbers, cauliflower, green peppers, spinach, baby carrots, broccoli, watermelon, strawberries, pineapple, cranberries, and oranges. When using fruit, be aware of the sugar content. If you're trying to lose weight, limit your serving size to a small amount.

4. **Healthy fats,** including nuts, seeds, avocados, coconut oil, avocado oil, MCT oil, and olive oil are the brain's preferred fuel source. Studies show that nutrients from fruits and vegetables are better absorbed when combined with fats—think salad with olive oil or broccoli with grass-fed butter or ghee or an apple with nut-butter. By adding healthy fat to your smoothie, you'll help with nutrient absorption and satiety. A tablespoon of nut butter or 1/4 of an avocado goes a long way.

5. **Fiber.** Most vegetables and fruits contain fiber. Fiber helps with digestion, and helps you feel full longer. Fiber aids in the body's detoxification process, removing toxins from the body. Fiber also helps slow the absorption of sugar into the bloodstream.

6. **Omega-3 fatty acids** from hemp seeds, avocado, coconut cream, chia and flax seeds, and strawberries are cancer-fighting, brain-boosting ingredients. Omega-3 fatty acids must come from the foods we consume and provide fuel for our brain.

7. **Nut milks** like almond, cashew, coconut, flax, and hemp provide a healthy dose of fat, protein, vitamins, and minerals. There are many nut milks on the market today. One of my favorites is from Califia Farms. Making your own almond milk is also a great option. It's easy to do, and

you don't have to worry about added ingredients. I would recommend not buying those with carrageenan, a common additive in nut milk used as a thickener and emulsifier to improve the texture. They also typically use this ingredient in ice cream, yogurt, cottage cheese, and processed foods. It can cause a host of problematic digestion issues.

8. **Herbs and spices,** such as ginger, turmeric, cinnamon, nutmeg, clove, mint, cilantro, parsley, basil, apple pie spice, and pumpkin pie spice. In addition to adding flavor, the antioxidants and anti-inflammatory benefits alone make these a great addition to your smoothie.

9. **Protein** from a high-quality protein powder, such as the Sunwarrior brand, hemp seeds, almonds, tahini, nut butter, pumpkin seeds, chia and flax seeds, oats, and dark leafy greens.

10. **Natural sweeteners** like dates, stevia, raw honey, maple syrup, coconuts, lemons, and limes. Most of the time, if you are using fruit, you won't need added sweeteners. You will find that after a while, your taste buds change, and the sugar in the fruit will be enough. Or use organic honey or maple syrup. But not agave nectar; agave nectar's manufacturing process makes it into a syrup, and it is 90 percent fructose. It has the same damaging effects as high-fructose corn syrup.

11. **Avoid any artificial sweeteners** like Splenda, NutraSweet, and Sweet 'N Low. Artificial sweeteners are made of toxic chemicals, cause major blood sugar spikes, make you crave more sugar, and cause visceral fat around the belly. Visceral fat is a form of gel-like fat that wraps around major organs, including the liver, pancreas, and kidneys. This dangerous

fat leads to diabetes, obesity, heart disease, stroke, cancer, dementia, and sleep disorders.

12. **Water.** Use filtered water, reverse osmosis, or distilled water, and avoid tap water. Tap water can contain chloride, lead, arsenic, and other harmful ingredients.

13. **Superfoods** like acai, aloe vera, cacao, spirulina, maca, goji berries, wheatgrass, and bee pollen. These superfoods are full of nutrients that your body craves. Using just one of these superfoods will help you get some serious nutrients into your body. All of the above are high in antioxidants and naturally support detoxification, and they are anti-inflammatory and have antiaging effects. Adding any one of these superfoods will have you feeling and looking your best.

14. **A note about dark leafy greens and thyroid issues:** If you are living with thyroid issues, raw, dark, leafy green vegetables contain glucosinolates, which can inhibit uptake and act as a goitrogen (goitrogens are substances that can suppress thyroid function). If people living with thyroid issues consume too much of these vegetables in their raw state, it will irritate their condition by creating a buildup of oxalic acid that can negatively affect the thyroid. I would suggest mixing up your vegetables using a light lettuce or celery and cucumber instead. When you use a mixture of vegetables and fruits, herbs, and spices, you'll get plenty of vitamins and minerals.

You may be wondering how to make a low-sugar smoothie when trying to lose weight? When making a smoothie, it is important to consider whether you are just maintaining your weight or if you are trying to lose a few pounds. If it is the latter, you will want to limit the amount of fruit you put into your smoothie. If you want to add some fruit, stay with the low sugar fruits, such as berries. I buy the organic strawberries, blueberries, and raspberries in the freezer section at the supermarket. That way you don't wait until they are in season and can enjoy them all year long. When watching added sugar, make up for sweetness by using fresh lemons, limes, and spices. Zesting the lemons and limes will add more sweetness too. Use spices like apple pie spice, cinnamon, cloves, nutmeg, and pumpkin pie spice to add more flavor. If you use an organic apple with cinnamon, you will feel like you're drinking a delicious apple pie, less all the added sugar and carbohydrates.

Create a healthy habit, making smoothies a regular addition to your meal planning. You'll crowd out the starch, sugar, and refined ingredient foods with this nutrient powerhouse. Play around with different ingredients. There are endless ways to make a smoothie. I have included a number of smoothie recipes in the back of the book in the Recipes Section.

The Scary Truth About Supplements

Most of us think that taking a multivitamin is the answer to staying healthy. The supplement world is unregulated, which means manufacturers don't have to go through the FDA approval process for effectiveness or safety. Many have harmful chemicals and toxic substances, such as GMOs, heavy metals (lead and arsenic), carrageenan, additives, and hydrogenated oils. And because supplements are not vetted by the FDA, they essentially place the burden for evaluating supplement safety, efficacy, and content labeling primarily on the shoulders of the manufacturers. With a smoothie, you know what you're getting—plenty of fiber, vitamin C, antioxidants, and immune-boosting vitamins and minerals.

Fruits and vegetables contain many biologically active ingredients that may help ward off illness and disease in ways that vitamins alone do not. A healthy diet is much more powerful than simply taking a daily multivitamin. When you're considering the pros and cons of multivitamins, consider what you expect to gain and why you think you need a supplement in the first place. If you need to supplement your diet because you're not eating well, vitamins are not going to be your answer. There's a reason why they call them "supplements." They should only supplement a healthy diet and cannot replace a healthy diet alone. Supplements can be expensive and, in most cases, aren't worth the investment. You will gain more with your money spent at the farmer's market or your local grocery store's organic produce section than with all of the supplements you currently purchase.

When using food for health, you know what you're getting. When using supplements for health, you need to know whom you're buying them from and if they are a trusted source. As I mentioned above, the FDA is not authorized to review these supplements for effectiveness or safety. It's important to defend yourself against poor quality supplements. There is a lot of confusion around purchasing the right supplements, as there are more than 90,000 vitamin and dietary products sold in the US. Most supplements have little to no data on their effectiveness. When looking to add supplements to my health protocol, I will seek out a Functional Medicine practitioner who supplies third-party-tested quality supplements (including probiotics). That way, I know I'm getting the highest quality supplements and don't buy the ones that are just wasting my money.

The counterfeit supplement world is a booming business. If you feel that you must purchase vitamins and supplements, you need to know where they are coming from. Alternative practitioners, such as chiropractors, acupuncturists, integrative practitioners, and Functional and Naturopathic doctors will do their due diligence in offering good quality supplements. There are thousands of counterfeit supplement companies that are eager to sensationalize their product and then take your money and run, so this will be your best route.

Gary Collins, who is a former special agent and forensic investigator for the FDA, has investigated fraudulent counterfeit supplement manufacturers and explains why it is not safe to purchase supplements from unknown, unreliable sources, including Amazon. In fact, Amazon is loaded with these unscrupulous supplement suppliers. Gary says:

> One of the easiest ways to make a dishonest buck in the supplement world is to create a pill that mirrors a name-brand health supplement. Create look-alike packaging, and you can sell your worthless pill on the internet for a "discounted" price. And a counterfeit operation is born!

When it comes to multivitamins, look at your diet first. Then, if your doctor sees you're deficient somewhere, you'll be able to make an informed decision and buy the right products. And when you're eating healthily, you'll also look to food for your daily dose of vitamins and minerals as well. Food is easier to digest and costs less. When you start looking at food as fuel for your body, you'll feel empowered to make healthy food choices, and you'll be excited to experiment with recipes to incorporate more of the colorful rainbow of fruits and vegetables versus disease-promoting, unhealthy foods, followed by your counterfeit multivitamin.

Remember, the easiest way to get a heavy load of vitamins and minerals every day is with smoothies. The powerhouse smoothie in the Recipes Section at the back of the book is full of vitamins, minerals, antioxidants, and immune-boosting fruits and vegetables that will keep you healthy. I've broken down each ingredient to help you see how you are fueling your body with vitamins, minerals, and immune-boosting health benefits.

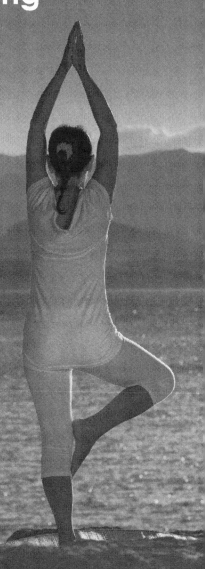

| SECTION 3 |

Understanding the Food You Buy

CHAPTER 13

Food Label Claims—
What Do They Really Mean?

"People are fed by the food industry, which pays no attention
to health, and are treated by the health industry,
which pays no attention to food."
— Wendall Berry

Determining the health quality of foods can be a daunting challenge and made more difficult by misleading food labels. Words like "free-range," "grass-fed," "natural," "organic," "hormone-free," and "gluten-free" seem to be everywhere these days. They appear on food packaging in the grocery store, usually in bold font followed by an exclamation point or listed on a menu at a restaurant. Many food labels can be confusing, so knowing what a food claim truly means is a great way to educate yourself about where your food comes from and how they produced it.

Marketers are smart, and they know we want food to not only taste good but to be natural and full of nourishing ingredients. At the same time, they care about keeping costs low and profits high. So they may throw in one organic ingredient and list organic on the label, but then the rest is filled with chemical preservatives, artificial sweeteners, and synthetic flavorings. Refer to the section on organic labels on page 154 to understand the organic guidelines.

When we can understand what food labels mean, we can begin to seek out as much real, whole foods as possible. This includes foods with a health claim on their package or those without any claim at all.

After you've mastered making proper food choices, it will become second nature, as you look for high-quality produce, meats, seafood, and prepackaged foods.

Grocery Store Produce SKUs

The following list will help you identify conventional, organic, and GMO produce at your local supermarket:

- Starts with "9" means it is organic
- Starts with "3" or "4" means conventionally grown
- Starts with "8" means genetically modified (GMO) or irradiated—AVOID!

Here is a list of common food labels and their brief descriptions:

"ANTIBIOTIC-FREE"

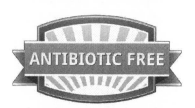

Antibiotic-free means that an animal did not receive antibiotics during its lifetime. Other phrases may say: "no antibiotics administered" and "raised without antibiotics."

Why should we be concerned about using antibiotics in farm animals? Antibiotic resistance is a widespread problem and one that the Centers for Disease Control and Prevention (CDC) calls "one of the world's most pressing public health problems." Bacteria that were once highly responsive to antibiotics have become more and more resistant.

The Consumers Union has concluded that the threat to public health from the overuse of antibiotics in food animals is real and growing. Humans are at risk, both due to the potential presence of superbugs in meat and poultry and to the general migration of superbugs into the environment, where they can transmit their genetic immunity to antibiotics to other bacteria, including bacteria that makes people sick.

According to the National Physician's Alliance:

As concerns about bacterial resistance and "superbugs" (like MRSA) increase and health professionals work to rein in the overuse of antibiotics in humans, the overuse of antibiotics in the production of food animals to promote growth and prevent illness in cramped, unsanitary living conditions is rampant and growing. As physicians, we can talk to our patients about antibiotic overuse and write fewer prescriptions, but we cannot solve this problem alone. We can't win the battle to preserve the effectiveness of antibiotics until meat producers are on board too.

Bottom line: Beware of commercial packaging that doesn't have a label at all. Those meats will most likely come from farm animals treated with antibiotics, due to the unsanitary conditions of their living spaces.

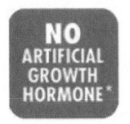 You'll see this claim in ads for chicken, turkey, pork, beef, and milk, as well as labels. One major reason it is misleading is that the US Department of Agriculture (USDA) doesn't allow farmers to feed hormones to poultry or pork—so there's no reason to choose products with this label. When you see this label on beef or dairy products, a third party hasn't verified it.

Buy certified organic meat, dairy, and poultry, which are free of both added growth hormones and antibiotics, or buy from small farmers whom you can ask about how they raise and medicate their animals.

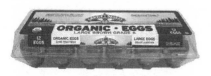

"CAGE-FREE" means they do not keep the hens that are laying the eggs in cages. They are free to roam inside a barn or warehouse, but generally, they do not have access to the outdoors.

What this doesn't explain is whether the birds lived outdoors in pastures or indoors in overcrowded conditions. If you are looking to buy eggs, poultry, or meat raised outdoors, look for a label that says "pastured" or "pasture-raised."

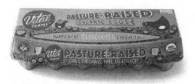

"PASTURE-RAISED" indicates that the animal lived and grazed on a pasture where it could eat nutritious grasses and other plants, rather than fattening up on grain in a feedlot or barn. Pasturing livestock and poultry is a traditional farming technique where they raise animals in a humane manner. Animals can move around freely and carry out their natural behaviors. This term is very similar to "grass-fed," though the term "pasture-raised" indicates more clearly that the animal lived outdoors in a natural environment.

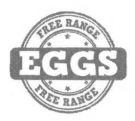

"FREE-RANGE EGGS AND POULTRY" The USDA only uses the terms "free-range" or "free-roaming" for egg and poultry production. The label can be used as long as the producers allow the birds access to the outdoors so that they can engage in natural behaviors. It does not necessarily mean that the products are cruelty-free or antibiotic-free or that the animals spent the majority of their time outdoors.

Free-range chickens have the opportunity to go outside. Smaller farms may keep birds outside under a canopy area. They may travel in and out of a barn at free will or spend some portion of their day roaming outdoors. There are no restrictions regarding what the birds eat. The USDA defines these terms, but third-party inspectors do not verify them.

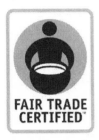

The **"FAIR-TRADE CERTIFIED™"** label means that farmers and workers, often in developing countries, have received fair wages and worked in acceptable conditions while growing and packaging the product. The Fair Trade Certified™ label ensures consumers that the farmers and workers behind the product got a better deal. It is more than a certification stamp and more than a seal of approval. It reassures consumers that their purchases are socially and environmentally responsible. It is the result of a rigorous global inspection and monitoring system.

According to Fair Trade USA, fair trade does promote organic farming with training for farmers and by offering a higher price for organic products. Many producers invest their fair-trade premium funds into organic certification, which has led to outstanding results: nearly half of all Fair-Trade Certified imports were also organic. They believe that in order to improve living and working conditions for farmers and workers, their environment must also be clean and healthy. Environmental standards are therefore integral to the fair-trade criteria. These include:

- Protecting water resources and natural vegetation areas
- Promoting agricultural diversification and erosion control (no slash-and-burn)
- Restricting the use of pesticides and fertilizers
- Banning the use of GMOs

All organic agricultural farms and products must meet the following guidelines (verified by a USDA-approved independent agency):

1. Abstain from the application of prohibited materials (including synthetic fertilizers, pesticides, and sewage sludge) for three years prior to certification and then continually throughout their organic license.

2. Prohibit the use of GMOs and irradiation.

3. Employ positive soil building, conservation, manure management, and crop rotation practices.

4. Provide outdoor access and pastures for livestock.

5. Refrain from antibiotic and hormone use in animals.

6. Sustain animals on 100 percent organic feed.

7. Avoid contamination during the processing of organic products.

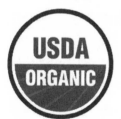 If a product contains the "USDA Organic" seal, it means that 95–100 percent of its ingredients are organic. Products with 70–95 percent organic ingredients can still advertise "organic ingredients" on the front of the package, and products with less than 70 percent organic ingredients can identify them on the side panel. Organic foods prohibit the use of hydrogenation and trans fats.

In order to be certified by the US Department of Agriculture (USDA), organic standards, farms, and ranches must meet a strict set of guidelines. A third-party certifier inspects the farms and ranches to ensure the organic standards are met and maintained.

***What about processed/packaged foods that contain the label:
"organic"? Are these a good choice?***

Walk down any aisle in the grocery
store, and you're sure to find a variety of
junk foods labeled "organic." Stores are
promoting more products like organic
cereals, organic candy, organic potato
chips, organic cookies, and organic crackers.

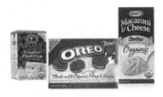

Surveys show that people are more apt to purchase a product with
the organic label on it because they perceive it to be a healthier choice.

If you see "organic" on the food label for chocolate chip cookies,
for example, it means that the main ingredients, such as wheat, sugar,
chocolate, and butter are cultivated organically. It doesn't mean that
the rest of the ingredients and nutrition profile of calories, fat, sugar,
and sodium in those cookies are any better than the regular chocolate
chip cookies sitting next to them. In addition, many organic junk
foods are made of highly processed ingredients, such as refined white
flour, sugars, salt, and oils with a ton of calories and sodium but not
much nutritional value.

How can we tell if a food labeled "organic" is a wise choice?

Read the label. If it has all kinds of claims on the front of the
package—beware. That is an advertisement for the product. Turn the
product over or on its side and read the label. That's where all the
ingredients are listed, including sodium, as well as important nutrients,
such as protein, fiber, and some vitamins and minerals. The ingredient
list includes all food ingredients in descending order by weight—if
you see highly refined ingredients, such as white flour, white rice, and
sugar appearing high up on the list, the product is probably a highly
processed food and has very little nutritional value. In addition, there

will be more ingredients; most of the time, you won't even know their meaning or be able to pronounce them. Those include artificial flavors, colors, sweeteners, and chemicals. That's when you can make an informed decision—to place the food product back on the shelf.

The Difference Between Organic and Non-GMO

Organic vs. Non-GMO

What do these labels really mean?	Organic	Non-GMO
No GMO ingredients	✓	✓
No artificial colors, flavors, or preservatives	✓	X
No synthetic fertilizers or sewage sludge	✓	X
No toxic, persistent pesticides	✓	X
No antibiotics or hormones for animals	✓	X
Animals eat 100% organic feed and pasture	✓	X
Protects wildlife and promotes biodiversity	✓	X
Enhances soil fertility	✓	X
Regulated by federal law	✓	X

Learn more about the benefits of organic!
www.ccof.org/why-organic

Both labels are different, and it is important to understand when picking out foods that are safe for you and your family. Because the non-GMO label is unregulated and can be produced alongside conventional products, packaged non-GMO foods may contain meat that has been raised on growth-promoting steroids and drugs, while organic animals aren't using antibiotics or growth hormones.

USDA Organic is regulated by the US Department of Agriculture. The organic label is a federal standard for how food is produced that requires a product to contain no GMO ingredients. This includes not only organic crops but meat as well: animals must eat only organically grown feed for their meat to be organic. Organic foods come with other benefits too—for instance, they can't be grown with synthetic chemicals or treated with irradiation.

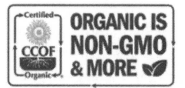

CCOF is a nonprofit organization that advances organic agriculture for a healthy world through organic certification, education, advocacy, and promotion. CCOF has recently created the above symbol to jointly signify both organic and non-GMO.

Bottom Line: Organic and USDA Organic is your best bet to avoid GMOs in your food.

What is the difference between "grain-fed" beef and "grass-fed" beef?

"GRAIN-FED"

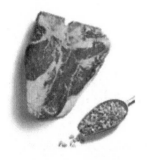

Animals raised on a grain diet are labeled "grain-fed." Large feedlots are called concentrated animal feeding operations (CAFOs). Here, the cows are rapidly fattened up with grain-based feeds, usually made with a base of soy or corn. These protein-rich grains help bring animals to market weight faster, and because they receive government subsidies, they are cheaper than other feed options. It has been estimated that the operating costs of factory farms would be 7–10 percent higher without these subsidies. As a result, a large percentage of grains grown in the US are used in animal feed: 47 percent of soy and 60 percent of corn.

"GRASS-FED" means the animals were fed grass, their natural diet, rather than grains. In addition to being more humane, grass-fed meat is more lean and lower in fat and calories than grain-fed meat. Grass-fed animals are not fed grain, animal by-products, synthetic hormones, or antibiotics to promote growth or prevent disease, although there may be times when they may have been given antibiotics to treat disease.

"FARM-RAISED" fish have been found to have high concentrations of antibiotics and pesticides. The crowded conditions of fish farms cause the fish to be more susceptible to disease. To keep them alive, farm owners administer antibiotics to the fish to stave off disease—

similar to what occurs in confined feedlot operations for cattle. In addition, farm-raised fish also have lower levels of healthy nutrients, 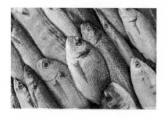 like omega-3 fatty acids. The omega-3 acids that are found in farm-raised fish are less usable in our bodies, compared to wild-caught fish. Farm-raised fish also has a lower protein content.

"WILD FISH" or "WILD-CAUGHT FISH" indicates that the fish was spawned, lived in, and was caught in the wild in their natural habitat. This is the ideal circumstance. When buying fish, you can find very helpful seafood guides on the Environmental Defense Fund website.[xxvii] In addition, the Monterey Bay Aquarium maintains a free list of the most sustainable seafood choices you can access with their Seafood Watch App for iPhone or Android.

Visit *www.MontereyBayAquarium.com* for more information.

"HORMONE-FREE"

The USDA has prohibited use of the term "hormone-free," but animals that were raised without added growth hormones can be labeled "no hormones administered" or "no added hormones."

Note: By law, hogs and poultry cannot be given any hormones.

Recombinant bovine growth hormone (rBGH) or recombinant bovine somatotropin (rBST) is a genetically engineered growth hormone that is injected into dairy cows to artificially increase their milk production. The hormone has not been properly tested for safety and is not permitted in the European Union, Canada, and some other countries. Milk labeled "rBGH-Free" is produced by dairy cows that never received injections of this hormone. Organic milk is rBGH free.

Fat-Free, Low-Fat, No Fat, Light, Reduced Calorie, oh my!

The FDA food labeling regulations require that essentially all food labels provide nutritional information to help consumers make informed food choices.

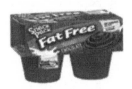

"FAT-FREE"

The "fat-free" or "no fat" definition is less than 0.5 grams of fat per reference amount and per labeled serving of a food. Less than 0.5 grams of fat per reference amount and per serving of food is considered a nutritionally insignificant amount of fat.

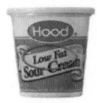

"LOW-FAT"

Low-fat means less than 3 grams of fat per serving.

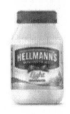

"LIGHT"

When a food label uses the term "light" or "lite," it indicates that a food has one-third fewer calories or 50 percent less fat (or 50 percent less sodium) than a comparable product.

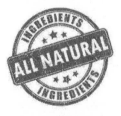

"NATURAL" means "minimally processed," and when you see this label, beware. No standards currently exist for this label, except when used on meat and poultry products. USDA guidelines state that "natural" meat and poultry products can only undergo minimal processing and cannot contain artificial colors, artificial flavors, preservatives, or other artificial ingredients. However, "natural" foods are not necessarily sustainable, organic, humanely raised, or free of hormones and antibiotics. A product that is labeled "natural" may very well contain GMOs.

The FDA, which regulates fruits, vegetables, and most processed foods, doesn't have a definition for the term "natural." So essentially, 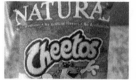 any food product can claim to be as "natural" as the manufacturer would like you to believe.

Bottom line: Foods labeled "all natural" are misleading. Opt for a better label, such as one that clearly states "antibiotic-free," "non-GMO verified," or "USDA Organic." Real food versus processed food is best.

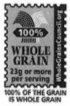 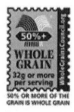 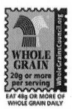

"WHOLE GRAINS"

The whole grain symbol appearing on the package was created by the grain industry, indicating the product has at least eight grams of whole grains per serving. This label implies that 100 percent of the grains used are whole. What it really means is a very small percentage is made with whole grains, added to many more refined grains. When looking for products using whole grains, make sure it says "100 percent whole grains" on the package. Finding these products may take a bit of investigative hunting at the grocery store, but the task is worth it to improve overall health. One hundred percent whole grains have more fiber and other nutrients than those that have been refined, a process that strips away the healthiest portions of the grain.

In addition, many whole grain foods are loaded with more carbs, sugar, and calories than we realize, and the government and food industry needs to come up with a better way to tell the consumer what's healthy and what's not.

What are Whole Grains?

There are a few foods that are always good sources of whole grain. The following list contains some foods that are guaranteed to be whole grain.

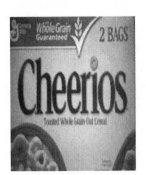

- Brown rice
- Bulgur wheat
- Oatmeal
- Popcorn
- Quinoa
- Barley
- Buckwheat
- Millet

When looking at a packaged product, ingredients are listed in proportional order so that the ingredients that are most used are listed first. Look for the words: "100 percent whole," as in whole wheat or whole grain. A trip down the bread and cereal aisles nowadays is nothing short of confusing for many consumers. These products, which boast jazzy marketing terms splashed across their packaging, often make it difficult for consumers to know if they're choosing wisely. Terms such as "whole grain," "multigrain," and "fiber" are on countless boxes and packages, but this doesn't always mean these products constitute a healthful and nutritious choice.

Even sugary cereals carry the whole grain stamp, which might lead consumers to think they're healthier than they really are. The whole grain stamp is one of the most widely recognized packaged food labels, and people think the foods are good for them, when—in fact—there are many other toxic ingredients at play.

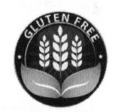

Gluten is a protein found in wheat, rye, oats, and barley. Gluten helps foods maintain their shape, acting as a glue that holds food together.

More and more grocery stores are stocking products labeled "gluten-free." It seems to be a

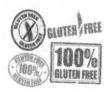

market that is exploding, and it's not because we are all living with celiac disease or have a gluten sensitivity.

Because "gluten-free" has become a popular catchphrase that implies the food is a healthier option, more products are marketing their claim to fame using "gluten-free" on their package. Beware of this trap, especially when it comes to processed food products. Inside that product is a host of nasty ingredients, most of which you won't even be able to pronounce.

How do we know if we are gluten intolerant?

Signs could look like:

- Abdominal bloating
- Fatigue
- Skin problems or rashes
- Unexpected weight loss or gain
- Joint pain
- Lack of focus/brain fog
- Memory problems
- Depression or anxiety
- Low immunity
- Hormonal imbalance and adrenal fatigue

A note on processed foods that have the gluten-free label: These foods will most likely have cornstarch, rice starch, potato starch, and tapioca starch used in place of wheat gluten, which causes extravagant blood sugar spikes and should be avoided.

To learn more about gluten, visit *http://www.celiac.org.*

Know your sugars! When a product is high in sugar but doesn't list sugar as a top ingredient on the label, beware. This means they may have disguised the sugar content cumulatively, using the combination of many forms of sugar. Various names of sugar include:

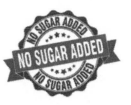

- Corn syrup solids
- Crystal dextrose
- Evaporated cane juice
- Fructose sweetener
- Fruit juice concentrates
- Malt syrup
- Maple syrup
- Molasses
- Concentrated fruit juice
- Hexitol
- Inversol
- Isomalt
- Maltodextrin
- Malted barley
- Nectars
- Pentose
- Raisin syrup
- High-fructose corn syrup

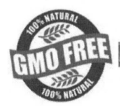 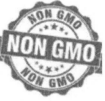 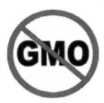

Genetically modified organisms (GMOs) are plants or animals that have been genetically engineered with DNA from bacteria, viruses, or other plants and animals. Products can be labeled "GMO-free" if they are produced without being genetically engineered using GMOs. First introduced into the food supply in the mid-1990s, GMOs are now present in the vast majority of processed foods in the US. The following chapter explains GMOs and their effects in detail. Read on to learn more!

Sources: *responsibletechnology.org, sustainabletable.org, humanesociety.org, ewg.org, foodandwaterwatch.org, celiac.org, nongmoproject.org,* and *ccof.org.*

CHAPTER 14

Why You Should Care About GMOs in Your Food

"Have genetically engineered (GE) crops contributed to the increased chronic disease burden in the US, especially in children? While the industry says 'no way', I believe the evidence suggests otherwise."
— Dr. Joseph Mercola, MD

What foods are genetically modified?

Currently commercialized GM crops in the US include:

- Soy
- Cotton
- Canola
- Sugar beets
- Corn
- Hawaiian papaya
- Zucchini
- Alfalfa

What type of GMO ingredients are hiding in our food?

The United States approved a host of GMO crops, ranging from apples and potatoes to GMO salmon (farm raised), which the FDA approved in late 2015 after long opposition from the public. New GMO crops get approval every year, and most GMOs on the shelves are unlabeled. Some may have a line on the label like "partially produced with genetic engineering," but that isn't required.

However, you're most likely to find GMOs hiding in the ingredient lists on processed foods. In 2014, 93 percent of corn and 94 percent of soybean acres in the US were GMO, and these crops sneak into your food in places you might not expect, from high-fructose corn syrup to sugar (made from sugar beets) to chemicals made from soybeans (used as additives in processed foods). Additives including cornstarch, corn meal, corn syrup, glucose, dextrose, canola oil, cottonseed oil, soy oil, soy flour, soy lecithin, and "protein extracts"— present in many processed foods—most likely derived from GMO crops. Livestock feed is also often made from GMO crops.

Other sources of GMOs:

- Dairy products from cows injected with the GM hormone rBGH

- Food additives, enzymes, flavorings, and processing agents, including the sweetener aspartame

- Meat, eggs, and dairy products from animals that have eaten GM feed

- Honey and bee pollen that may have GM sources of pollen

- Some of the genetically modified ingredients are: vegetable oil, vegetable fat, and margarine (made with soy, corn, cottonseed, and/or canola)

GMOs are making the news nearly every day, and issues surrounding their safety are a source of ongoing controversy. Roundup, for example, can cause sterility, hormone disruption, birth defects, and cancer. They engineer most GMO crops to be herbicide tolerant. Monsanto sells "Roundup ready crops" designed to survive applications of Roundup herbicide. This very process means you are consuming dangerous chemicals when you eat genetically modified foods.

In addition, genetic engineering creates dangerous side effects. The genetically modified plants can result in massive collateral damage that produces new toxins, allergens, carcinogens, and nutritional deficiencies.

Up to 80 percent of the packaged foods sold in grocery stores today contain GMOs, but you wouldn't know it because products containing them don't require labeling. More consumers are GMO-aware, so now the Non-GMO Project Verified label has surfaced and is the fastest-growing label in the natural products industry.

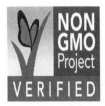 Non-GMO products are in demand and the Non-GMO Project Verified seal is the most trusted non-GMO label among consumers. This label gives shoppers the assurance that a product has completed a comprehensive third-party verification for compliance with the Non-GMO Project standard.

When it comes to food labeling, third-party certifications are best because they ensure the claim is unbiased, rigorous, and transparent.

The Non-GMO Project Product Verification Program is North America's only third-party verification for non-GMO food and products. Third-party verification is the highest quality system when it comes to product labeling and certifications because it ensures products have been comprehensively evaluated by an independent party for compliance with a standard developed by industry experts and stakeholders.

Companies must work with third-party technical administrators to get their products verified.*

Although a food labeled "non-GMO" may be a better choice, if you really want the superior product, shop local at your farmer's market or look for the USDA Organic label. If a product has USDA Organic seal that means all of the ingredients used are 100 percent organic.

Preserving and building the Non-GMO Project Verification and USDA Organic supply chain is a critical step toward transitioning to a safe, healthy food supply for future generations.

Source: non-gmoproject.org

In an effort to educate you further on the importance of avoiding GMOs, I am including an article written by Cynde Christie. Cynde is a personal friend of mine and has done an amazing job researching the health effects of consuming products that have been genetically modified. She explains this complex process in a clear, concise manner. I hope you find this information helpful and informative:

Most people who have heard of GMOs want to avoid them. Not everyone actually knows what a GMO is, but people generally know that they are bad. So, let us take a brief look at what a GMO is, why they developed them, and how they are used, and then, I will tell you how to keep them out of your life.

GMO stands for "genetically modified organisms." Take an organism, such as corn; insert a gene of another organism into the corn, and you have modified it into a GMO. For example, one of my personal favorites: putting spider DNA into goat milk when making bulletproof vests strong like spider webs. Unfortunately, there are currently no regulations for safety testing on genetically modified organisms.

Genes make up all living things within their DNA. Most living things, animal and vegetable, have a natural ability to fight off the intrusion of alien genes. This means that the GMO scientists must take very drastic measures to force the genes from two different species together into one organism. These measures include using viruses and bacteria to invade animal or vegetable genes, injecting genes into other genes, and other, equally frightening and frankly draconian methods. A couple of examples of the "blending" used in GMOs are: Arctic fish genes injected into tomatoes and strawberries for tolerance to frost, and human genes inserted into corn to produce spermicide. Nowadays, vegetarians have to be really on their toes to make sure that they are actually eating only vegetable matter!

The general school of thought for the scientists when developing GMOs was that they were good for increasing food production and helping plants to become more pest-resistant. The problem was that in making those two seemingly beneficial things happen, many negative aspects resulted. The nutritional value of the food diminishes due to cell disruption. The result is that we have food with little nutritional value, riddled with poison but a much bigger profit margin. Also: "super weeds!" Super weeds are weeds that are so pesticide resistant, they require stronger and stronger pesticides to keep them at bay. Glyphosate, a systemic pesticide that is soaked up inside the plants that the animals and we eat, is the primary pesticide used on GMO crops today. The main component of Roundup is glyphosate. They breed many GMO crops to be "Roundup ready," meaning that they can withstand multiple sprayings of pesticide. That means more Roundup sales. The result is that humans are eating more of and stronger pesticides (poison) that has become endemic in their lives. Once again, the economy drives science.

On the human side, the scientific meddling has resulted in more and stronger allergens in children and adults that are harder to treat. More children are developing autism than ever before. This is just a small example of the many human costs associated with GMOs.

The currently commercialized GMO crops in the US include soy (94 percent), cotton (90 percent), canola (90 percent), sugar beets (95 percent), corn (88 percent), Hawaiian papaya (more than 50 percent), zucchini, and yellow squash (over 24,000 acres). Any food that contains these ingredients most likely have some degree of GMO, and these plants are designed to tolerate pesticides.

According to *Mother Earth News*, other products that are heavily GMO include dairy, eggs, meat, cookies, snacks, chips, ice cream, frozen prepared meals, oils, fats, shortening (except olive oil), condiments, prepared foods, bread, and crackers. Many of these fall into the GMO category due to ingredients used in preparation or feed ingredients for animals and poultry. The more ingredients listed on the packaging of a processed food, the more likely it is that it contains GMO components.

Now for the good news, GMO food items are not that hard to avoid. Here is how:

1. **Buy organic.** By law, Certified Organic foods cannot contain pesticides or fertilizers or genetically engineered seeds.

2. **Non-GMO certifications.** There are now Non-GMO verified programs that test products to verify whether they contain any GMO material. This certification program will not approve any food product if it contains more than 0.9 percent GMO content. A new certification, the GMO Guard Verification Program from Natural Food Certifiers, is a stricter testing program that will not certify anything with more than 0.05 percent GMO material. These certifications appear as labels on non-GMO food products.

3. **Do not buy nonorganic frozen, processed (boxed or canned) premade meals.** Most all of them are, to some extent, GMO products.

4. **Join a CSA.** Community sustained agriculture (CSA) groups are in most areas where people have the ability to grow food. You pay a fee that the farmers use as seed money, and then every week or so during the growing season, you receive a box of whatever is fresh that week. CSAs are a wonderful thing!

5. **Shop at a farmer's market near you.** Farmer's markets are everywhere, and you can buy fresh produce directly from the farmer.

CHAPTER 15

Pulling It All Together

Knowledge Is Power

You've made it! It is my hope that you have gained a lot of useful knowledge and information about how important it is to achieve optimal health as you move through the third stage of your life. The lifestyle modifications presented in this book, if followed according to your own individual needs, will dramatically improve your overall health and wellness. You now know you don't have to become a slave to a cookie-cutter diet plan or continue with a yo-yo dieting path that, in the long run, ages you more. If you follow the whole food nutrition approach outlined in this book, you'll not only lose the weight, you'll feel more energized, gain your health back, and feel and look amazing! Replace the bad with the good, one by one, and you'll see extraordinary results!

Learn to Be Adaptable Without Judgment

Understand that it's a day-by-day choice, and things arise that sometimes can be out of our control. Life is not always perfect. With your new awareness, you can begin to know that one minor setback is just that. Your new lifestyle doesn't control you—you control it. People with highly restrictive diet plans inevitably fall off the wagon, give in, and go back to their old ways. Then their confidence plummets. You will no longer fall into that trap. Nor will you judge whether you're good or bad when you realize that you are just human, and you will show yourself the love and compassion you deserve as you nourish your mental, emotional, physical, and spiritual well-being. Remember to embrace that inner child in you who stills needs love. That love is so precious and can only come from within.

You're the CEO of Your Health Plan

You now realize that you can be your best doctor, and that it's vital to tap into that intuition toolbox that resides within. You have the courage and awareness to see things differently now and feel more in control than you ever have in the past. You realize that Western medicine does wonders for treating acute trauma, surgeries, and cutting-edge therapies that save lives, but it has a long way to go when addressing preventive care. That's where you come in. Your knowledge will enable you to become your own health advocate. Our healthcare system needs a major overhaul when it comes to treating chronic illness and disease, and your gift is the knowledge that there is a better way, by looking at prevention versus simply managing symptoms with medications. Seek out a Functional Medicine practitioner who will help address the root cause of your health issue and find supporting practitioners, such as a health coach, nutritionist, acupuncturist, masseuse, etc.

Prioritize Your Healing Efforts

You now know how important it is to heal from past wounds, trauma, and negative lifestyle choices. Now is your time to heal. Healing can happen at any given moment when you have a *burning desire* to want a better way. Seek out support to help you process your pain as you focus on your healing journey. Set yourself as the number one priority now! Don't waste another moment suffering. Days turn into weeks and weeks turn into months, and before you know it, your life has passed, and you haven't fully lived it. You deserve more joy, more happiness, more love, and more compassion. Your own inner work has to happen before your outer world aligns with your true desires.

Your Personal Blueprint

The information presented in this book is a blueprint. Do what works for you and what aligns with your personal preferences. Your personal blueprint may be different, yet it will have the same core values (a healthy diet, exercise, self-care, etc.). Choose the healthy foods that make sense to your personal taste, work schedule, budget, and cultural ideals, whatever matters to you most. You'll design the perfect lifestyle that fits your needs and gain more knowledge as you do so. Your health payoff does not come from one single recipe or food group; it comes from continually being mindful of eating healthily with a mix of real foods over a long period. Your central awareness around practicing self-care plays a major role as well.

Heal Your Gut Microbiome

Your gut health is the hub of your immune system and also establishes communication to your brain. You now know that a diet rich in whole, unprocessed foods will encourage the growth of good bacteria in the gut, helping to establish a strong immune system. The role of gut microbes in the immune system are affected by modern lifestyle, diet, and overuse of antibiotics, causing an increasing disruption of the gut microbes that stimulate the immune system. Chronic inflammation is linked to most chronic illnesses that begin with dysfunctional gut microbiota. As new science emerges, you'll see more awareness and information addressing this important issue in conventional medicine, as well as Functional Medicine.

Address Hormonal Imbalances

After reading the chapter on weight-loss resistance and hormonal imbalances, you'll have a better understanding of how hormones play a major role in your overall health, and uncover the reason why you can't lose weight as you enter your menopausal years. Too many women suffer through hormonal symptoms without investigating the areas where they may be out of balance, causing uncomfortable symptoms, such as mood swings, hot flashes, low energy, brain fog, etc. Seek out a healthcare practitioner (see Chapter 7) who can help you with diagnostic testing to pinpoint the hormonal imbalances and then take steps to rebalance them in a way that alleviates your symptoms so you can have a better quality of life.

Rejuvenate Your Body Now for A Healthier Tomorrow

After reading this book, you have a better understanding of why you do not want to neglect your body with a sedentary lifestyle. A sedentary lifestyle is a contributing factor to chronic illness or disease. Our bodies are meant to move! When we start taking care of our most important vessel, our body, we not only look and feel amazing, our bones benefit, our mood lifts, and our energy levels soar. Exercise triggers the release of "feel-good hormones," or endorphins, in the brain. If you suffer from back pain, don't underestimate the importance of strengthening your core! Your core strength will help lessen and sometimes eliminate overall pain. I know it worked for me. Living with scoliosis, degenerative disc disease of my spine, and osteoporosis, I make it a priority to strengthen my core with exercises such as yoga, Pilates, and strength training. Before I implemented these steps into my daily practice, I suffered chronic, severe pain, and my course of treatment was pain medications and other drugs to help control my symptoms. Those medications came with multiple side effects and led to a low quality of life. I don't have to be a patient for life anymore because my understanding grew about how important it is to stay strong and keep my body working to its full capacity.

Remember, *the more you take care of your body, the more your body takes care of you!*

Rewrite Your Life Story

Finally, the language that you use is either fueling or sabotaging your well-being. Pay attention to your thoughts, emotions, and self-talk. Whether you're conscious of your language or not, your self-talk will determine what's truly inside your heart. If that language is working against you, find the courage to seek a new perspective. Staying the victim is a dead-end road. You can easily course correct and drive down the road that empowers you to seek new answers. Those people who don't give up will find a better way, and there is always a better way. Feeling overwhelmed, scared, uncertain, or resentful is a sign that there's work to do. It's easier to take the path of least resistance when we're feeling this way. That's when we settle and hand over our power to the circumstance or the person who is robbing us of our energy. Acknowledge that the situation or actions of another person hurt you deeply. Take action to protect your physical and emotional well-being. Learn to honor and love yourself unapologetically. Staying silent will harden your heart, dampen your spirit, and disconnect the spinal cord to your truth. You can teach yourself to become a warrior of truth. That will set you free from emotional and physical pain. Use this affirmation: "I will focus on surrounding myself with positive people and things that lift me up, and disregard the rest."

There is nothing more beautiful than loving yourself completely; deep contentment will rise above any obstacle that comes your way. When you're happy, joyful, and satisfied with how you manage your life, you'll have the freedom and the courage to express yourself fully. You'll discover time to play more, to laugh more, and to find inner peace.

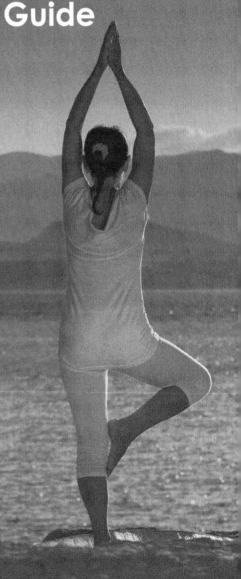

SECTION 4

Reference Guide

Easy Health Management

The following guide is to help you make the changes in your diet and lifestyle easy to implement, and you can refer to this information often with an at-your-fingertips guide.

First, I will explain about the environmental toxins that we all need to avoid, followed by some of the lists of foods to include and/or introduce in your new healthy lifestyle.

Additionally, I have included the following for your convenience:

- Information on local and organic vegetables and their benefits.

- The "21-Day Sugar Reduction Anti-Inflammatory Diet Guide" helps you take steps to eliminate pro-inflammatory foods and replace them with healthier options.

- A healthy five-day workweek meal plan provides an example for you to follow, and I have included those recipes, as well as a few of my favorites, for you to enjoy.

- Time-Saving Tips for Eating Healthily During the Work Week.

- I have included a document titled: "Your New Health Mindset Checklist." This will be a great resource for you to print out and keep handy as you start your new health journey.

- The Environmental Working Group's (EWG) "Dirty Dozen and Clean 15" produce list helps when you're produce shopping.

- Finally, I have put together a list of websites, books, videos, and audio programs that I often refer to as a reference tool, and I want the same for you as you embark on your new health journey!

Remove Environmental Toxins from Your Home

Below are some helpful recommendations and steps you can take to gain health, by removing exposure to environmental toxins. Environmental toxins are cancer-causing chemicals and endocrine disruptors.

1. **Don't drink tap water.** Drink plenty of clean, filtered water instead. Reverse osmosis filtered water or distilled water is best. Tap water has a host of ingredients that are toxic. Drinking the right water helps detoxify your body and keeps you hydrated. Avoid plastic bottles that leach toxic chemicals, such as BPA, into your body. Use glass or metal bottles instead. To find out the safety of your area's water supply, visit the Environmental Working Group's website *https://www.ewg.org/tapwater.*[xxxviii]

2. **Replace toxic chemicals from your home,** including skin creams, makeup, nail polish, deodorant, cleaning products, and soap with organic, safe alternatives. There are so many dangerous chemicals lurking inside these products ranging from:
   - **Formaldehyde** (a known Class A carcinogen used as a disinfectant, fixative, germicide, and preservative in a wide variety of products, from deodorants to liquid soaps to nail varnishes to shampoos.)
   - **Parabens.** If the product you are using contains methylparaben, ethylparaben, propylparaben, butylparaben, and isobutylparaben, it has parabens. They are added to deodorants, toothpastes, shampoos, conditioners, body lotions, and makeups to stop the growth of fungus, bacteria, and other potentially damaging microbes. Parabens disrupt hormone function, an effect linked to

an increased risk of breast cancer and reproductive toxicity.

- **Phthalates** can be found in shampoos, shower gels, hairsprays, and top-selling perfumes and nail varnishes. Animal studies have shown phthalates can damage the liver, kidneys, lungs, and reproductive system—especially developing testes.
- **Sodium lauryl sulphate (SLS)** SLS can be found in many shampoos, bubble baths, liquid soaps, etc. It is a known skin irritant, stops hair growth, and can cause cataracts in adults and damage children's eye development. The lure to the consumer is that it's cheap and produces many bubbles.
- **Toluene** is in nail enamels, hair gels, hair sprays, and perfumes. It is a neurotoxin and can damage the liver, disrupt the endocrine system, and cause asthma.
- **Talc** is carcinogenic and has been linked to an increased risk of ovarian and endometrial cancer and general urinary tract disorders.
- **Xylene** (also listed as xytol or dimethylbenzene) in nail polish bottles. This can damage your liver.
- **Parfum/perfume:** fragrances have been linked to allergies and breathing difficulties.
- **Dangerous Ingredients in Cleaning Supplies:** There are too many ingredients to mention and when in doubt, purchase from a safe source such as Method, Seventh Generation, and Tropical Traditions. Refer to the Think Dirty App and EWG's Healthy Living App (link on the following page).

There are hundreds of more dangerous chemicals lurking in your home. The easiest way to track which products are safe or not is with the following two apps; you can use to look up the safety of your products.

The first is Think Dirty *https://www.thinkdirtyapp.com*[xxix] and the second is EWG's Healthy Living App. *https://www.ewg.org.*[xxx]

Additional food sources that have dangerous chemicals and toxins in your home include:

3. **Heavy metal exposure.** Reduce your intake of high mercury fish, such as tuna, mackerel, swordfish, and Chilean sea bass. Limit these, and when looking for a healthier option, use wild-caught salmon.

4. **Beware of food labels disguised as being healthy.** Don't rely on a food product's health label. So far, the food industry is doing an outstanding job of tricking us into believing that many food products in our grocery store aisles are health food. Refer to my chapter on food label claims.

When you see a health claim, it means there are many nasty ingredients inside that container, and the food product is highly processed and loaded with chemicals and industrial seed oils that all cause inflammation in our body. The FDA allows this junk food into our food supply. These products promote cancer growth, obesity, and ill-health, yet are disguised as a healthy option. If the food product has a health label—beware! Kale, avocado, and brussel sprouts don't require labels! It's a crazy and insane world where our food industry can get away with this kind of madness. When I saw a certain cheese labeled gluten-free, I thought to myself, "Cheese doesn't contain gluten." However, a "cheese-like product" that is made to taste like cheese, with artificial ingredients, chemicals, and dyes, does! Knowledge is power, now more than ever. We don't have to become a victim of our food supply! When we get educated on what to look for, we stop purchasing food that is making us sick.

5. **Avoid numbers.** No ingredient on any box or package should have a number, such as Red No. 40 or Yellow No. 6. These are toxic chemicals. The Center for Science in the Public Interest (CSPI) says food dyes pose some risks to the American public and is calling on the FDA to ban Yellow No. 6. Yellow No. 6 contains known carcinogens and contaminants that unnecessarily increase the risks of cancer, hyperactivity in children, and allergic reactions. You will find this in processed foods, including the popular Ritz Crackers.

6. **Avoid processed foods, excessive sugar, sugary soft drinks, pastries, white flour, etc.** All of these products promote obesity and poor health. They are loaded with processed ingredients, chemicals, and dyes. Refer to my Weight Loss Chapter on ways to crowd out these problematic foods and incorporate nutrient-dense whole foods to promote health, not disease.

7. **Beware of industrial seed oils.** Soy, canola, corn, peanut, sunflower, safflower, and cottonseed oil all fall under the term "vegetable oils," making them sound like a healthy option. Why wouldn't they? The word "vegetable" makes you think of kale, broccoli, and spinach. However, what the word "vegetable" here really means anything that is not an animal. In addition, 90 percent of soy and canola oils are genetically modified. The rise of seed oils has contributed to chronic disease and has changed the composition of the American diet with the intake of processed foods. Seed oils contain high amounts of a type of fat called omega-6 PUFA. Omega-6 fats are chemically less stable than other types of fat, such as olive oil, coconut oil, avocado oil, and clarified

butter. When these problematic oils are exposed to heat, light, or oxygen, they create oxidative stress in the body. These oxidized fats are highly inflammatory to the body and create chronic inflammation. And inflammation is yet another reason to eliminate these types of oils, as well as the processed foods that contain them.

- **Remove unhealthy staple options and replace with healthy ones.** Remove sugar in all its forms. Include anything with the words "agave" or "high-fructose corn syrup." Remove artificial sweeteners. (Use stevia, monk fruit, honey, or maple syrup instead)
- **Refined flours, white flour, white bread, and white pasta.** (Use almond meal, coconut flour, brown rice pasta, and sprouted bread instead)
- **Canola oil, soybean oil, vegetable oils, or hydrogenated oils.** (Replace them with coconut oil, ghee, avocado oil, and olive oil)
- **Processed breakfast cereals.** (Replace them with smoothies, eggs, and avocados)
- **Margarine or butter replacements.** (Use butter or clarified butter instead)
- **Any food product that includes preservatives, flavorings, colorings, or thickeners.**
- **Conventional meats and eggs.**
- **Any farm-raised fish (including shrimp)** These fish live in unsanitary conditions and contain pesticides
- **Processed deli meat.** Avoid meat that contain nitrates. Sodium nitrate increases the risk of cancers, diabetes, and heart disease. Butylated hydroxyanisole (BHA) and butylated hydroxytoluene (BHT) are possible carcinogens.

Nourishing Foods to Include:

1. **All dark, leafy greens.** Kale, collard greens, broccoli, spinach, mustard greens, Swiss chard, arugula, Brussel sprouts, and romaine lettuce are your cancer-fighting soldiers!

2. **A rainbow of fruits and vegetables.** Include carrots, tomatoes, beetroots, eggplants, mushrooms, dark leafy greens, cranberries, lemons, limes, oranges, strawberries, blueberries, raspberries, and blackberries, and red, green, yellow, and orange peppers. They contain the highest amount of a beneficial compound called phytochemicals that help boost their cancer-fighting ability.

3. **Tree nuts.** Include almonds, pecans, hazelnuts, walnuts, Brazil nuts, macadamia nuts, and pistachios. Including a handful twice daily helps keep blood sugar in check and works towards the prevention of diabetes and insulin resistance. Nuts are an antioxidant powerhouse!

4. **Seeds.** Seeds come in a wide variety and offer multiple nutritional benefits from fats, minerals, fiber, protein, and antioxidants. The seeds I recommend are flax, chia, hemp, pumpkin, and sesame. The omega-3 fatty acids in flaxseeds help reduce inflammation. Keep your serving size the same as nuts, at a handful or two a day.

5. **Healthy fats.** Clarified butter, coconut oil, olive oil, avocado oil, grass-fed meat, fatty fish, nuts, and seeds.

6. **Good-quality protein.** Grass-fed beef and antibiotic- and hormone-free chicken, turkey, pork, and wild-caught fish. Legumes (if tolerated) and pasture-raised eggs. The best plant proteins that are both complete and highly bioavailable are:

- Spirulina
- Hemp
- Soy
- Quinoa

- Lentils
- Buckwheat
- Amaranth

Herbs and spices to fight illness, including cancer:

- Cinnamon
- Turmeric
- Ginger

- Garlic
- Cayenne pepper
- Oregano

Additional Things You Can Do

Juicing

According to the Gerson Institute, "Fresh pressed juice from raw foods provides the easiest and most effective way of providing high-quality nutrition. By juicing, patients can take in the nutrients and enzymes that are easy to digest and absorb." This cancer-fighting protocol suggests you juice daily.

Smoothies

Smoothies are another great way to get in your green and colorful fruits and vegetables! The difference between juicing and making a smoothie is with a smoothie, the fiber is still readily available from the vegetables and fruits, whereas juicing strips it out. You can also add in things like chia, flax and hemp seeds, loose-leaf matcha green tea, spirulina, nuts and seeds, and other superfoods.

Local and Organic Vegetables

Some types of conventionally grown produce are much higher in pesticides than others are, and it is good to avoid them. Others are low enough that buying non-organic is relatively safe. *The Environment Working Group's (EWG)* "Annual Shopper's Guide to Pesticides in Produce"™ lists the Dirty Dozen™ fruits and vegetables with the most pesticide residues and the "Clean Fifteen"™, for which few, if any, residues were detected.

When buying organic produce is not an option, use the "Shopper's Guide" to choose foods lower in pesticide residues.

The following fruits and vegetables have the highest pesticide levels, so they are best to buy organic. They are known as the "Dirty Dozen":

- Apples
- Sweet bell peppers
- Cucumbers
- Celery
- Potatoes
- Grapes
- Cherry tomatoes
- Kale/collard greens
- Summer squash
- Nectarines (imported)
- Peaches
- Spinach
- Strawberries
- Hot peppers

Fruits and vegetables that you can buy conventionally grown, known as the "Clean 15." These conventionally grown fruits and vegetables are generally low in pesticides.

- Asparagus
- Avocados
- Mushrooms
- Cabbage
- Sweet Corn
- Eggplant
- Kiwis
- Mangos
- Onions
- Papayas
- Pineapples
- Sweet peas (frozen)
- Sweet potatoes
- Grapefruit
- Cantaloupes

For an annual updated list, go to *www.ewg.org*.

The 21-Day
Sugar Reduction
Anti-Inflammatory Diet Guide

The following guide is going to help you reduce inflammation and oxidative stress from common food sensitivities, inflammatory fats, processed carbohydrates, added sugar, and food chemicals. It's a simple replace-this-with-that guide to show you how to nourish your body with high-quality protein, cruciferous vegetables, healthy fats, fiber, and quality nutrition, while eliminating pro-inflammatory foods.

By eating this way, you'll learn to support the digestive tract and boost your immune system and liver with key nutrients, antioxidants, and bioflavonoids to allow optimal detoxification and blood sugar balance. This will help you realize which foods may be causing you problems, from weight gain to low energy to brain fog. Every symptom that shows up is due to something in your diet that is not agreeing with you. You can print this guide and use it as an easy reference when you are meal planning or simply looking for a snack.

It's important to note that not all the foods on the left will be bad for you. But, the only way to know which foods may be causing you inflammation is to eliminate them for a period of time, then reintroduce them to see which trigger foods are causing you discomfort.

You'll gain the knowledge to take action and change some of your eating habits that will benefit your health, energy, and vitality!

Foods to Eliminate	Foods to Add
Dairy products: Milk, cheese, cream, yogurt, butter, and nut butters.	Low-sugar, unsweetened, almond, coconut, or cashew and milk or clarified butter (ghee).
Grains: Anything containing wheat, gluten, (including whole grains and processed foods made from grain flour).	We eliminate all grains for twenty-one days to determine if they are contributing to inflammation. After that, you can add in whole grains such as brown rice, wild rice, and quinoa.
High glycemic foods and fruit, including anything with added sugar. • Flour • Rice • White potatoes • Some fruits: bananas, grapes, cherries, watermelon, apricots, mangos, and papaya • Raisins, dried fruit • Bread • Breakfast cereal	Low glycemic fruits: • Raspberries • Blackberries • Blueberries • Strawberries • Lemons • Limes • Green apples

Foods to Eliminate	Foods to Add
Sugary drinks, including sweetened coffees, sodas, fruit juice, and energy drinks.	Water, carbonated water, coffee (black), tea, and herbal tea.
Peanuts Canola oil*, soy oil, corn oil, and vegetable oil.	Raw almonds, sesame seeds, pumpkin seeds, walnuts, clarified butter, coconut oil, and extra virgin olive oil.
Eggs, soy,* soybeans, and soy products (to discover if you have a sensitivity and the GMO factor). Legumes: If they cause gas and bloating, avoid them. If not, use as a healthy protein and carbohydrate option.	Replace soy milk with almond, cashew, or coconut milk.
Processed deli meats, hot dogs, and bacon. (Much bacon has added sugar, so eliminate it for now.)	High-quality protein: • Grass-fed beef • Hormone- and antibiotic-free chicken, turkey, and pork • Wild-caught fish (The best option is to cook a whole chicken or turkey breast and use it throughout the week. When this is not possible, a safe option is Applegate Organics products, available in your grocery store refrigerator section.)

1. *In the United States, over 90 percent of canola oil is genetically modified. Canola oil is a refined oil that's often partially hydrogenated to increase its stability, but this increases its negative health effects.

2. *The vast majority of soybeans, 87 percent, are genetically modified.

Healthy Meal Plan Example

	Breakfast	Snack	Lunch	Snack	Dinner
DAY 1	Cinnamon/ Pear Green Smoothie (double up for a snack in the afternoon)	1/4 c. Mixed Raw Nuts	Chicken Vegetable Soup (prepared on weekend)	Cinnamon/ Pear Green Smoothie	Ratatouille with Chicken (weekend prep)
DAY 2	Berry Overnight Oats (double up for leftovers snack or breakfast other days)	Apple with Nut Butter	Leftover Ratatouille w/Chicken	Berry Overnight Oats leftovers	Cauliflower Ground Beef Bake (time-saving tip: prepare ground beef on weekend)
DAY 3	Protein Pancakes	Cut Up Veggies with Hummus	Leftover Chicken Vegetable Soup Or Leftover Cauliflower Ground Beef Bake	Chocolate Chia Pudding (make extra for next day)	Shephard's Pie (ground beef already cooked, boil and mash cauliflower for topping (Can all be done ahead of time)

Healthy Meal Plan Example
(continued)

	Breakfast	Snack	Lunch	Snack	Dinner
DAY 4	Green Eggs	Chocolate Chia Pudding	Dill Salmon Salad	Roasted Chickpeas (batch cook for next day's snack)	Roasted Chicken (Chicken prepared on weekend) with steamed broccoli. Add brown rice or quinoa* (batch cook these in Instant Pot over a weekend)
DAY 5	Strawberry-Banana Smoothie	Hard-boiled egg with sliced avocado	Chicken Lettuce Wraps (using leftover chicken from whole chicken dinner)	Roasted Chickpeas	Mediterranean Chickpea Salad w/ Leftover Chicken Vegetable Soup Or Your choice of leftovers from this week's menu

*If you have a large family, double up on the chicken, cook two instead of one, and use all the leftovers during the week for lunch, dinner, and snacks. You can even freeze leftover cooked chicken to use the following week.

For recipes, see the Recipes Section.

Time-Saving Tips for Eating Healthily During the Work Week

Here are some timesaving tips to help you plan and eat healthily throughout the week. Eating healthily doesn't have to be hard, it just has to be a priority!

1. Set aside three to four hours on Saturday or Sunday, so you have enough time to go grocery shopping, familiarize yourself with ingredients and prepare foods to eat later in the week, and wash and pre-chop veggies and snacks.

2. Precut snacking veggies like celery, carrots, turnips, bell peppers, cucumbers, etc., so you always have something you can easily grab out of the fridge. Store them in a covered dish with a little water to keep them from drying out. It's a lot easier to make a good choice if you have good choices readily available. Dip them in a little tahini, hummus, or black bean dip for a quick and nutritious snack.

3. Make one snack recipe and one sweet treat recipe so you have these ready to go when you're feeling tired or have a craving.

4. If time is short in the mornings, make double batches of smoothies or breakfasts that are easy to grab and go.

5. Make a big pot of greens that are ready to go anytime by setting a pot of water to boil. Clean and de-stem the greens, then tear them into bite-sized pieces. Once the water is boiling, drop in the greens, turn off the heat, and cover—let sit for two minutes. Drain, rinse with cool water, and store in the fridge. Blanched greens will keep for about a week in your fridge.

6. Set up a salad bar in your fridge. Make a few salad dressings to last you the five days. If you wash a bunch of lettuce, greens, precut cucumbers, celery, radishes, carrots, green onions, and anything else you like, you'll be able to build a salad in no time. These foods stay fresh for about three days in the fridge when precut. When you plan, you are investing in your most important asset—yourself!

Your New Health Mindset Checklist

Here are my top reasons why I believe you can maintain health when you have the knowledge to choose your foods wisely and take care of your physical and emotional well-being. I have addressed all of this information previously in this book but have put this list together for easy reference.

✓ You deserve to take time for yourself and nurture your emotional, physical, and spiritual well-being.

✓ You can relieve your symptoms and get to the root cause of your health issue by using a Functional Medicine approach. (Refer to Chapter 4.)

✓ You can find health at your local grocery store, farmer's market and local, sustainable farms.

✓ You can learn how to make smoothies that will help build a healthy immune system. (Refer to Chapter 12 and the smoothie recipes in the back of this book.)

✓ You can rely on your inner doctor to call out when a certain health protocol, given by your current physician, is not working.

✓ You can build strong bones and pain-free joints by knowing which foods to eat to help you maintain healthy bones. (Refer to Chapter 10.)

✓ You can have less colds and viruses when you eat foods that will nourish your body, not deplete your body.

✓ You can have a healthy glow when you eat a rainbow of fruits and vegetables, and eliminate fake, processed foods and incorporate more collagen (including bone broth) into your diet.

✓ You can improve your energy levels and feel sexy and alive through a healthy diet, daily exercise, and practicing self-care.

✓ You can realize that the cheap food product substitutes will offer chronic disease on a silver platter.

✓ You can have the confidence to ignore the latest fad diet and know which foods are good versus the foods that promote ill-health.

✓ You can have a healthy pH, which promotes health. Knowing whether foods are acidic or alkaline is easy and as simple has referring to Chapter 10 on building healthy bones.

✓ You can get off the dieting roller coaster when you remove simple (bad or refined) carbohydrates in the form of pasta, bread, pastries, white sugar, white flour, white bread, some whole wheat breads, muffins, crackers, chips, sweetened soft drinks, fruit juices, etc.

✓ You can stop cancer in its tracks! You can quit your sugar addiction, and you must! Excess sugar causes inflammation, and inflammation feeds cancer cells. Consider this: Cancer cells love glucose and have up to nineteen times more glucose receptors than normal cells.

✓ You can learn what's in a healthy plate: protein, vegetables, whole grain/starches (brown rice, quinoa, sweet potatoes, and squash), and healthy fats (olive oil, coconut oil, and grass-fed ghee).

✓ You can control your sugar cravings by sipping on herbal tea or almond milk with vanilla, eating a few pieces of dark chocolate (75% or higher) or a bowl of berries, sweetening with stevia and cocoa, and eating a snack high in protein (nuts and seeds).

✓ You can do an elimination diet to see which foods are causing you discomfort. Refer to Chapter 7 on weight loss challenges or get an IgG food sensitivity test from your doctor.

✓ You can start an exercise routine, including weight bearing exercises that will nourish your body and mind as you move through your new health journey.

✓ You can limit negative energies from your life without feeling guilty. You deserve this!

✓ You can go gluten- and dairy- free. These two food groups cause the most inflammation and side effects including anemia, osteoporosis, skin rashes, joint pain, irritability, nasal congestion, sinus infections, bloating, and gas.

✓ You can start addressing your emotional wounds, negative energies, and past trauma, and seek out healing practitioners to help you process your pain in order to heal and move on with your new life. (Refer to Chapter 3.)

✓ You can seek out a Functional Medicine practitioner or endocrinologist to help with hormonal imbalances. You do not have to suffer through menopause! There are things you can do to alleviate your symptoms and address imbalanced hormones and the metabolic and metabolism changes that take a hit during menopause. Refer to Chapter 7, the section titled "The Role of Hormones."

✓ You can buy organic meats. A few online sources are: *www.butcherbox.com*[xxxii] and *waldenlocalmeat.com/what-is-a-share.*[xxxiii] Avoid conventional meats. Buy local, organic, grass-fed, and antibiotic- and hormone-free chicken, turkey, and pork, and wild-caught fish. Grass-fed beef is lower in overall and saturated fats, higher in omega-3s, contains up to four times as much Vitamin E, and is higher in CLA—a nutrient associated with lowering cancer risk. Conventional meats are grain-fed and are fattier with more calories. Grass-fed cattle are free-roaming, live outside, and graze on grass or hay, while grain-fed are fattened with grain that is hard to digest, and treated with hormones, antibiotics, and additives to speed their growth. Many conventional chicken ranchers feed their poultry arsenic! This is another reason to buy organic.

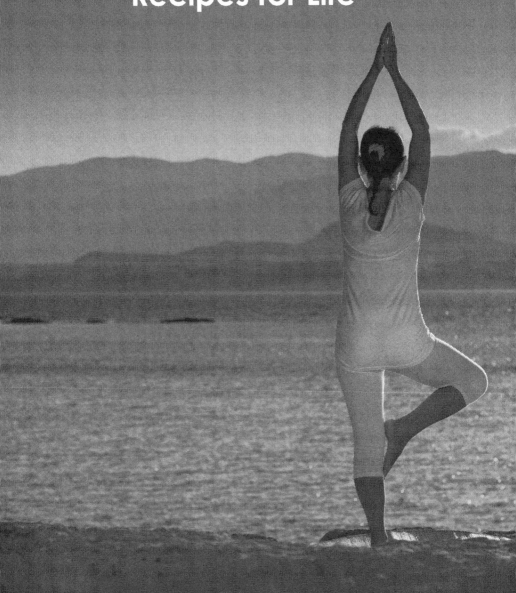

| SECTION 5 |

Recipes for Life

Have Fun Recipes

I am not a chef. I learned to cook my own meals because I want to be healthy. Simplicity is key. Here are some easy recipes. The recipes with a star are on the Healthy Meal Plan, and all of these recipes are gluten-, dairy-, and soy-free. And by all means, have fun creating your own!

BREAKFAST

Paleo Powerhouse Breakfast

Scrambled eggs, bacon, spinach, tomato, and basil recipe

Ingredients:

3 c. of spinach, kale, or Swiss chard*
1/2 c. of organic grape tomatoes, chopped in half
1/4 c. prepared pesto (olive oil, garlic, and chopped basil)
6 pasture-raised, organic eggs
2 Tbsp. avocado oil
6 slices of organic turkey bacon or organic pork bacon
(no nitrates, hormones, or antibiotics added)

Directions:

1. Place greens and tomato in a pan with avocado oil, sauté 3–5 minutes.
2. Place the bacon in a separate pan and cook until done.
3. Whisk together eggs with some water, salt, and pepper to taste.
4. Add eggs to pan with greens and tomato.
5. Add about 2–3 Tbsp. of pesto mixture.
6. Remove bacon from pan, cut into small pieces, and add to eggs.

Note: If you would like, double this recipe. You can have leftovers for the rest of the week.

Note: *More supermarkets are offering prepackaged, organic greens. Stop & Shop's Nature's Promise brand offers its Organic Power Blend, which has organic kale, red chard, spinach, collard greens, frisée, and mizuna. This is a wonderful way to add more greens without having to purchase them separately.
Serves 2–3

---

*My Favorite Green Power Smoothie
Put in your Vitamix (or your blender):
1/4 c. cilantro (or parsley)
2 celery stalks
3 large kale leaves
1 green apple
1 lemon—zest lemon and use juice
1/2 tsp fresh or ground ginger
1/2 tsp fresh or ground turmeric
1/2 ground cinnamon
1/4 tsp organic vanilla
3 c. of almond milk
1 or 2 scoops of Sunwarrior Protein Powder
3 Tbsp. organic flax or chia seeds
Water with ice
Serves 1

Seed Porridge with Fresh Berries
Ingredients:
2 Tbsp. unsweetened coconut flakes
1 Tbsp. raw pumpkin seeds

2 tsp chia seeds

1 Tbsp. cacao powder

1 Tbsp. raw flax seeds

1/2 c. fresh strawberries, raspberries, or blueberries

1 scoop of protein powder

2–4 Tbsp. nondairy (coconut, almond, hemp, etc.). milk

Directions:

1. Grind the first 3 ingredients together and cover with 4–6 oz. hot water.
2. Allow to sit for 5–10 minutes or until chia seeds have gelled to create a porridge. Grind flax seeds separately, and then add to porridge with milk and fruit.

Serves 1

---

*Strawberry-Banana Smoothie

Ingredients:

1 small banana

2 Tbsp. chia seeds

2 Tbsp. nut butter

1/2 c. frozen organic strawberries

8 oz. coconut, almond, hemp milk, or water

1 small handful of fresh spinach or kale

1–2 scoops Sunwarrior Vanilla Protein Powder

Directions:

1. Place all ingredients into a high-speed blender. Start blender on low, and increase speed to combine fully.
2. If you don't have a high-speed blender, start by blending the fruit, chia seeds, nut butter, and liquid together until smooth. Then add the greens and blend again.

Serves 1

*Protein Pancakes

Ingredients:

2 medium ripe bananas

2 eggs, slightly beaten

2 Tbsp. almond butter

1 tsp vanilla

1/4 c. coconut flour

Coconut oil for cooking

Directions:

1. Using a fork, mash banana in a medium size bowl. Then add egg, almond butter, vanilla, and coconut flour, and stir until combined.
2. Heat a medium skillet over medium-high heat. When warm, add coconut oil and swirl to coat skillet. When the oil has melted, scoop some of the pancake mixture into the pan and cook until set and browned on one side. Then flip, and cook until browned on the other side. Remove from pan.
3. Serve with a little real maple syrup or fresh fruit.

Serves 1

Blueberry-Banana Smoothie

Ingredients:

1 c. frozen or fresh organic blueberries

1 small banana

1 c. almond or coconut milk

1 c. chopped spinach, collard greens, or kale

1 Tbsp. freshly ground flax seeds

1–2 tsp raw honey

2 scoops of Sunwarrior Vanilla protein powder (20g)

1–2 scoops organic collagen protein powder

Directions:

Combine all ingredients in a blender and blend until smooth. It helps to start at a low speed and slowly increase speed as the ingredients begin to blend. Add water by the quarter cup, if your smoothie needs a little more liquid.

Serves 1

Daily Multivitamin Smoothie

(There's a lot here. This makes approximately four servings. Its purpose is to show you how much antioxidants, vitamins, minerals, fiber, protein, and fat you're getting from using whole foods.)

1 c. chopped kale	(High in vitamins C and K, and revs up the body's detoxification process.)
1/2 c. alfalfa sprouts	(High in vitamins C and K, antioxidants, and omega-3 fatty acids, it helps build strong bones, prevents iron deficiency, and is nutritionally dense and very low in calories, with loads of fiber.)
1 c. chopped bok choy	(Includes powerhouse vitamins C, A, K, plus calcium, magnesium, potassium, manganese, and iron. Great for cardiovascular health.)
1 Tbsp. chopped cilantro	(Removes heavy metals, lowers blood sugar, and is anti-inflammatory.)
1/2 zucchini	(Rich source of B vitamins; boots energy.)
1 carrot	(Rich in antioxidants; helps with acne and skin problems.)
1/2 avocado	(Healthy fat and high in potassium; lowers "bad" LDL cholesterol.)

1 c. pineapple	(High in vitamin C and antioxidants; supports immune system and digestion.)
1 c. blueberries	(High in antioxidants; reduces inflammation and oxidative stress.)
1/2 c. strawberries	(High in vitamin C, antioxidants, fiber, and potassium.)
1 banana	(High in potassium; helps maintain fluid levels in the body.)
1 lemon, juiced	(High in vitamin C, digestion, and hydration; cleanses the cells.)
1 Tbsp. shredded coconut	(Antibacterial; boosts immune function).
3 scoops collagen protein	(Supports bone health and is a protein source.)
2 tsp spirulina superfood	(Powerful antioxidant and anti-inflammatory, it can lower "bad" LDL cholesterol and triglyceride levels, and contains vitamins B1, B2, B3, copper, and iron.)
2 tsp flax-chia seed blend.	(Includes fiber and omega-3s.)
1 Tbsp. ground cocoa powder	(A superfood: Containing more antioxidants than blueberries, cocoa is one of the richest sources of polyphenols. It's especially abundant in flavanols, which have potent antioxidant and anti-inflammatory effects.)
2 c. almond milk	(Protein)
2 c. of water	(Hydration)
Ice	(Hydration)
Serves 4	

Kicking Cancer's Butt Kale Smoothie

Ingredients:

1 c. coconut water

1 c. kale

1/2 green apple

1/4 avocado

1/2 cucumber

1/2 lemon (zest and juice)

A handful of cilantro

1 scoop Sunwarrior Vanilla Protein Powder

Water and ice for consistency

Directions:

Add all the ingredients to the blender, except water.

Check consistency and add water if needed.

Serves 1

---

*Cinnamon/Pear Protein Smoothie

Ingredients:

1 ripe pear, seeded

1 Tbsp. ground flax seeds

2/3–1 c. almond milk

1/4 tsp cinnamon

1/4 tsp raw honey

1 small handful spinach, kale, or collard greens (stems removed)

1 scoop Vanilla Sunwarrior Protein

1/2 c. ice cubes

Directions:

1. Combine all ingredients in your blender. Turn your blender on low and increase speed until all ingredients are incorporated.

Serve immediately.

2. Tip: If you don't have a high-speed blender, smoothies often blend better if you blend all of the fruit with the liquid first. Then add the remaining ingredients, and blend again.

Serves 1

---

*Berry Overnight Oats

Ingredients:

1/2 c. rolled oats

1/2 c. mixed frozen organic berries (raspberry, blueberry, strawberry, blackberry, or whichever ones you have on hand)

1 Tbsp. chia seeds

1 c. coconut, cashew, or almond milk

1/2 Tbsp. maple syrup (optional)

Directions:

1. Combine all ingredients in a bowl first. (If doubling this recipe, it's easier to put in the bowl first, mix, then transfer to a small mason jar or glass container with a tight-fitting lid.)
2. Place in refrigerator overnight, and enjoy the next morning.

Serves 1 (double the recipe if you want leftovers)

---

*Green Eggs

What a great way to get more greens into your breakfast! You can batch cook this recipe, and use muffin tins for a grab-n-go breakfast or snack idea!

Ingredients:

2 eggs

1 c. fresh spinach or baby kale (rinsed and dried)

1 Tbsp. chopped cilantro (or herb of choice)

1 small clove garlic, minced

1/2 tsp sea salt

1 Tbsp. coconut or avocado oil

Directions:

1. Combine eggs, greens, cilantro, garlic, and salt in a blender until combined.
2. Place oil in small skillet to coat plan.
3. Heat over medium, and then add egg mixture and cook for 3–4 minutes, turning frequently until set.
4. Add salt and pepper to taste. Then serve.

Serves 1

LUNCH

Salmon, Arugula, and Sweet Potato Salad

Ingredients:

1 small sweet potato, scrubbed and cut into small chunks

1/3 lb. wild salmon fillet, seasoned with salt and pepper

2 Tbsp. white wine vinegar

2 tsp Dijon mustard

2 Tbsp. olive oil, divided

1/4 c. finely chopped chives (optional)

10 oz. arugula, washed

Sea salt and freshly ground pepper

Directions:

1. Heat oven to 450 degrees. Place sweet potatoes on a rimmed baking sheet and toss with 1 Tbsp. olive oil. Season with salt and pepper, then roast for 10 minutes, tossing occasionally.
2. After 10 minutes, toss the sweet potatoes again and move to the side of the baking sheet. Place salmon on the other side and roast for 8–10 minutes until salmon flakes easily. Remove from oven and let cool for 5 minutes.

3. Meanwhile, place vinegar, Dijon mustard, and remaining oil in a small bowl and whisk together. Season with sea salt and pepper. Place arugula in the bowl, and toss to coat with the dressing.

4. Top with salmon and sweet potatoes, and then serve.

Serves 1

*Dill Salmon Salad

Ingredients:

1 6–8 oz. can wild salmon (drained) or 6-oz. cooked wild salmon

1/2 Tbsp. capers, drained

1 Tbsp. finely chopped red onion

2 Tbsp. hummus

1 Tbsp. olive oil

2 Tbsp. rice wine vinegar

1 Tbsp. fresh dill (chopped) or 1–2 tsp dried dill

3 c. salad greens, rinsed and dried

2 Tbsp. raw sauerkraut (optional)

Sea salt and freshly ground black pepper to taste

Directions:

1. Combine salmon, capers, onion, hummus, oil, vinegar, and dill in a large bowl and mix well.

2. Add salad greens and toss to combine.

3. Season with sea salt and pepper, and if using sauerkraut, place on top. Enjoy!

Serves 1

*Spicy Roasted Chickpeas
(Paleo: You can do this with raw cashews as well!)

Ingredients:

2 (15-oz.) cans chickpeas/garbanzo beans

2 Tbsp. avocado oil

1/4 tsp ground cumin

1 tsp smoked or regular paprika

Pinch cayenne pepper

1 tsp sea salt

Directions:

1. Preheat oven to 400 degrees.
2. Rinse and drain chickpeas. Make sure you dry them well: place them in a towel or paper towel and roll to dry. Then place them in a medium bowl.
3. In a large bowl, whisk together avocado oil, cumin, paprika, cayenne, and sea salt. Add chickpeas, and toss until evenly coated.
4. Line baking sheet with parchment paper. Spread the chickpeas in a single layer on a baking sheet, and bake for 30–35 minutes (or until golden brown and crispy). Halfway through, shake the tray to flip the chickpeas for a more even bake.
5. Remove from oven, and place in a serving bowl or airtight containers for later use (up to three days).

Serves 1 (increase amount to have more for later)

---

*Chicken Lettuce Wraps

Ingredients:

1 Tbsp. olive oil

1/2 tsp paprika

1/2 tsp cumin

1/2 tsp sea salt

Leftover chicken from whole chicken

3 large leaves of lettuce (Boston, butter, or romaine)

1 mango, peeled and cut into long strips

1/2 avocado, peeled and cut into long strips

1/2 red pepper, cut into long strips

1/4 c. chopped cilantro

Lemon or lime wedges for serving

Directions:

1. Heat skillet to medium-high heat.
2. In a small bowl, mix together oil and spices.
3. Slice leftover chicken meat into thin strips, and add to oil and spice mixture.
4. Coat and cook for 2–5 minutes until heated.
5. Meanwhile, arrange lettuce leaves on a plate. Place chicken, mango, avocado, and bell pepper inside the leaf; then top with cilantro.
6. Squeeze fresh lemon or lime over the top of each one.
7. Roll each leaf closed to enjoy as a wrap.

Serves 1

---

*Mediterranean Chickpea Salad

Ingredients:

1 14-oz. can chickpeas/garbanzo beans, drained and rinsed

1/2 c. cucumber, chopped

1/2 c. cherry tomatoes, chopped

1/2 c. red bell pepper, chopped

1/4 c. Kalamata olives, pitted and chopped

1 Tbsp. fresh oregano (chopped) or 1 tsp dried

1 Tbsp. fresh dill (chopped) or 1 tsp dried

1 Tbsp. apple cider vinegar

2 tsp Dijon mustard

1 Tbsp. olive oil

1 tsp sea salt

1 tsp freshly ground pepper

3 c. salad greens, washed and dried

Directions:

1. For dressing: In a small bowl, whisk together apple cider vinegar, Dijon mustard, olive oil, oregano, dill, salt, and pepper.
2. Place salad greens in a large bowl, and top with chickpeas/garbanzo beans and chopped vegetables. Start adding dressing to the mixture, and taste as you go, adding more or less, depending on your taste buds.

Serves 2

Chicken Vegetable Smash—Gluten and Dairy-Free

Ingredients:

Leftover bone-in chicken breast meat, shredded

One zucchini (spiralized)

1 c. mushrooms of choice, chopped

1-16 oz. bag Cascadia Farms Organic Mixed Vegetables (for a quick recipe or cut up your own)

Two small stocks of bok choy, rinsed and chopped

8 oz. chicken bone broth (homemade or use Kettle & Fire brand)

1/4 c. gluten-free flour, sifted

1 Tbsp. ghee

2 Tbsp. avocado oil

Salt and pepper to taste

Directions:

1. Spiralize zucchini in spiralizer—set aside.
2. Heat oil in pan, and cook mushrooms and bok choy for 5 minutes.
3. In a small 2-quart pan, put 1/3 c. of water in with frozen mixed vegetables; cook 7–9 minutes.

4. Transfer spiralized zucchini to the pan with mushrooms and bok choy. (Zucchini will cook when you place broth in the pan and heat up the dish.)

5. Place shredded chicken in the dish and mix with vegetables.

6. In a separate pan, heat chicken bone broth with 1 Tbsp. ghee. When boiling add 1/3 c. of gluten-free flour of choice; heat and whisk until smooth. If you still have some lumps, you can transfer it to your blender and blend well.

7. Pour the broth over chicken and vegetables, and cook for 5 minutes. Serve or save for later.

Serves 4

---

*Donna's Golden Chicken Vegetable Soup (Crockpot)

Ingredients:

One package of organic, antibiotic- and hormone-free chicken thighs (4–6 pieces)

Or 1 pack of organic, antibiotic- and hormone-free chicken drumsticks (6–8 pieces)

4 (organic) celery stalks, chopped

4 (organic) carrots, chopped

2 c. of green beans, chopped

2 c. of frozen organic peas

One onion chopped or sliced in half (to remove later)

Two cloves of garlic, chopped

3 c. cauliflower rice (prepared) or long grain brown rice

1 c. chopped spinach

1/4 c. chopped parsley

1/4 c. chopped basil

2–3 Bonafide Bone Broths (are now sold at Whole Foods Market) or 4–5 Kettle & Fire Bone Broth (or use your own homemade bone broth)

1 Tbsp. apple cider vinegar

One pinch of rosemary and thyme

Sea salt and pepper to taste

16+ oz. of water

Directions:

1. Cut onion in half and place on bottom of a Crock-Pot.
2. Place chicken thighs or drumsticks on top of the onion.
3. Add apple cider vinegar to top of chicken. (This pulls out the nutrients from the chicken bones.)
4. Add in celery, carrots, green beans, peas, and garlic.
5. Cook brown rice (or cauliflower rice) according to instructions and set aside.
6. Hold off putting rice (or cauliflower rice), spinach, parsley, and basil into the pot until the last hour of cooking.
7. Add in the bone broth.
8. Add water to the top of the pot.
9. Add sea salt and pepper to taste.
10. Add rosemary and thyme.
11. Put Crock-Pot on high for one hour.
12. Then put on low for 7 hours.
13. Halfway around 3–4 hours, remove chicken, let it cool, peel the chicken off the bone, break it down to string-like pieces with a fork, and save it for later. (You will add the chicken back at the end.) In the meantime, put chicken bones back into the soup to get all the nutrients from the bones. Remove bones once the pot is done.
14. At hour 7, add in rice, spinach, parsley, basil, and chicken.

Serves 6

*Easy Paleo Broccoli Soup

You can make this broccoli soup recipe in as little as 15 minutes. This soup is rich and creamy with a hint of garlic. There is no need to use heavy cream, like traditional broccoli soups. Instead, I use full-fat coconut milk and grass-fed ghee to add a rich, creamy texture and flavor. Then blend all of the ingredients in your Vitamix to make this soup smooth and delicious.

Ingredients:

1 extra-large head of broccoli

2 cloves garlic, peeled

4 c. chicken stock or vegetable stock

1 Tbsp. grass-fed ghee

1 c. full-fat coconut milk

Sea salt to taste

Fresh ground pepper to taste

Directions:

1. Bring broccoli, garlic, chicken stock, and coconut milk to a boil over medium-high heat. Cover, reduce heat, and simmer for 10 minutes.
2. Carefully transfer to Vitamix and puree until smooth (or puree with an immersion blender).
3. Add ghee, salt, and pepper, and blend to combine.

Serves 2

Tomato-Eggplant Soup (Dairy-Free)

Ingredients:

4 Tbsp. of avocado, coconut, or olive oil

1 medium-to-large eggplant, sliced and then cut into quarters

2–3 large garlic cloves

2 large in-season beefsteak tomatoes, cut up into quarters

10 grape tomatoes, cut in half

1 zucchini, sliced into 1-inch thick chunks

1 onion, chopped

2 carrots (or 10 baby carrots), cut into small pieces

2 celery sticks, chopped

1 c. chopped basil

1 c. chopped parsley

6 c. of chicken broth or stock

1 can diced tomatoes

2 Tbsp. of tomato paste

Salt and pepper to taste

Directions:

1. Preheat oven to 400 degrees.
2. In a large bowl, combine zucchini and eggplant in oil and place on a lined baking sheet, and bake for 1/2 hour.
3. In a separate deep skillet, add the rest of the oil and sauté onion and garlic on low-medium heat for 3–5 minutes.
4. Add one cup of chicken broth.
5. Add beefsteak and grape tomatoes.
6. Add diced tomatoes and tomato paste.
7. Add basil and parsley.
8. Sautee for 1/2 hour.
9. Add eggplant and zucchini to stew and sauté for another 20–30 minutes.
10. Fill a Vitamix, blender, or food processor with stew and 1 cup of chicken broth.
11. Blend to make a cream-like soup. It will take approximate 3–4 times to use all of the ingredients.
12. Garnish with fresh, cut up basil and serve.

Serves 3–4

Beeting Your Cold Soup

Ingredients:

2 whole beets, cut up into small chunks

1 c. organic strawberries

3 pieces of kale or 1 c. of chopped kale

2 Tbsp. honey

1/4 c. coconut milk

2 c. of water

Directions:

1. Blend all ingredients in a Vitamix, high-powered blender, or food processor until smooth.
2. Place in the fridge for one hour; serve chilled.

Serves 2–3

Simple Cabbage and Bok Choy Recipe

If you double up on this recipe, you may have leftovers for lunch the following day or two. It only takes about 20 minutes, including chopping the cabbage and bok choy and sauteeing it in the pan. This recipe is a gluten-free option.

Top it off with some brown rice or cauliflower rice along with your protein of choice to make a delicious and satisfying meal.

Time-saving Hint: On Sunday, roast a few bone-in chicken breasts or a whole chicken or sausage, or saute some grass-fed ground beef or ground turkey to use during the work week. Then add to a dish like this, and your meal is done!

Time-saving Hint: Make your rice in bulk; then either put it into the refrigerator to use that week or freeze in containers and pull them out in the morning to defrost, heat, and serve at night. When I make my rice in bulk, I use my Instant Pot. (It's another Sunday prep item.)

Cabbage and Bok Choy Stir-Fry

Ingredients:

1/4 head green cabbage, cut into thin ribbons

3 baby bok choy or 1 small bunch regular bok choy, rinsed and sliced into small strips

1/2 c. shredded carrots (time-saving tip: purchase prepackaged)

1 Tbsp. wheat-free tamari

1 Tbsp. rice wine vinegar

2 tsp toasted sesame oil

1 tsp red pepper flakes (optional)

1 Tbsp. sesame seeds (optional)

Directions:

1. Heat a large skillet to medium-high heat.
2. Add cabbage and 1 Tbsp. water, and sauté for 2–3 minutes, tossing occasionally.
3. Once the cabbage has started to wilt, add bok choy (sliced stalk first, then leaves), carrots, wheat-free tamari, and rice wine vinegar.
4. Continue sautéing until the cabbage, bok choy, and carrots wilt. Then turn off heat and add sesame oil, red pepper flakes, and sesame seeds. Serve immediately.

Serves 2

DINNER

Roasted Garlic Mashed Cauliflower
(Instead of Mashed Potatoes)

Ingredients:

One or two cauliflower heads (make more to use during the week)

1 Tbsp. of ghee

Salt and pepper to taste

2 cloves of garlic

2 Tbsp. avocado oil (good for high smoke point)

Directions:

1. Preheat oven to 350 degrees.
2. Cut up cauliflower into florets.
3. Drizzle garlic with avocado oil and place in small ceramic dish with lid; bake for 15 minutes.
4. Place cauliflower in a pan with water using steamer insert, and cook for 15-20 minutes or until tender.
5. Mash cooked cauliflower, garlic, and ghee in a large bowl using an immersion blender.
6. Place cauliflower in a casserole dish and bake for 15 minutes, allowing flavors to blend.

Garnish with salt, pepper, and parsley.

Serves 2–3

Shrimp with Zucchini, Summer Squash, Sweet Potato, and Rutabaga Noodles (Instead of Pasta)

All you need is a spiralizer to make these great noodles. Depending on what vegetable you are using, it only takes a few minutes, sautéing in olive oil, to cook. Add basil, tomato, and garlic for a scampi-style dish. In this case, I used cooked shrimp, but you can use steak or chicken as well.

In addition, if you have your favorite home-cooked spaghetti sauce, add a pound of ground meat or chicken, and you are good to go!

Serves 2

Cauliflower Rice

This rice, made from chopped cauliflower, will boost your fiber and nutritional value and leave you more satisfied after your meal. If you haven't tried making cauliflower rice before, you'll love the mild flavor.

Another option is to purchase riced cauliflower, prepackaged in the grocery store refrigerator. There are so many reasons why making cauliflower rice is good for you. You're able to eat more vegetables, add volume without calories, and bulk up dense dishes without added carbs!

Directions:

1. Place cauliflower chunks in a food processor or Vitamix and pulse until broken down into rice-size pieces.
2. Heat avocado or coconut oil in a skillet over medium heat.
3. Add rice cauliflower, salt, and pepper.
4. Cover skillet and cook until heated through (3–5 minutes).
5. Remove lid and fluff rice with a fork.

Note:

Add chopped onion, spices, and fresh herbs to this dish to bring out more flavor.

Serves 2–3

---

*Sausage and Vegetable Ratatouille for the Slow Cooker

The Crock-Pot is my number one cooking tool to use when making soups, stews, and dishes like this one, to have on hand in my fridge when I lose track of time and still want a healthy meal. It saves time during the week and goes a long way.

Ingredients:

1-3 uncooked sausage, chicken, or pork (remove casings and crumble)

1 large green and red bell pepper

1 medium eggplant

1 zucchini

1 summer squash

1 c. mushrooms (white button, cremini, or similar)

3 Roma or heirloom tomatoes

1 large yellow onion

2 carrots

3–4 medium cloves garlic, crushed or finely chopped

1 c. chicken broth* (see notes)

1 25-ounce jar pasta sauce* (see notes)

pinch of kosher salt

1/2 tsp of black pepper

Fresh basil (or parsley) for serving

Directions:

1. Slice bell peppers in half, remove seeds, and cut into 1-inch pieces.
2. Trim ends off eggplant, slice in half, and then cut into 1-inch cubes.
3. Trim ends of zucchini and summer squash, slice in half, and then cut into 1-inch cubes.
4. Slice tomatoes and cut in half.
5. Slice mushrooms in half, depending on size. Larger: slice twice, then half.
6. Chop onion in half, then into small pieces.
7. Slice carrots into small pieces.
8. Crush garlic using a garlic press (or finely chop).
9. Finely chop basil or parsley to sprinkle when serving.
10. Pour 1 c. of broth into a pot, followed by remaining ingredients.

Hold the tomato sauce and crumbled sausage for last. Combine all ingredients in the Crock-Pot, mix well, cover, and cook on high for 4 hours (or on low for 7 hours).

Notes:

Making bone broth from scratch is best. Make ahead, freeze, and pull out when needed. If you don't have homemade broth on hand, I also use Bonafide from Wise Choice Market (also available at Whole Foods Market). They make it from scratch from all organic ingredients. It is full of nutrients, and you can drink it in place of coffee or tea as well. *www.wisechoicemarket.com/.* Another great option is Kettle & Fire brand, which you can find at Whole Foods Market or *http://www.ThriveMarket.com.*

Pasta sauces can have added sugars, sodium, and other nasty ingredients, so you want to pay attention to the label. There should be no more than 4 grams of sugar per serving. Great options include Monte Bene, Dave's Gourmet Organic, or Michaels of Brooklyn with only 4 grams of sugar per serving, very low sodium, and no cornstarch or MSG.

Serves 4–6

---

*Cauliflower and Ground Beef Bake

Ingredients:

1 Tbsp. avocado oil

1 onion, diced

1/2 Tbsp. of minced garlic

1 lb. ground beef (or turkey)

1 head of cauliflower, chopped into florets

1-24 oz. marinara sauce, without added sugar

(I use Dave's Gourmet Organic Roasted) Garlic and sweet basil

1 can crushed tomatoes

Salt and pepper to taste

1 cauliflower

Directions:

1. Heat the oil in a large skillet, and sauté the onions 3–5 minutes until translucent.
2. Add minced garlic and ground meat and sauté until browned, stirring to crumble the meat (add salt and pepper to taste). Add tomatoes and marinara sauce to meat.
3. In a separate pan, spread the cauliflower florets in a large baking dish.
4. Pour the meat mixture over the cauliflower.
5. Cover the dish, and bake at 350 degrees for 45 minutes.

This dish goes a long way, and you'll have plenty left over for another night or lunch the next day.

Note: You could add cut up cooked sausage to this dish to add more flavor.

Serves 4–6

Chicken Bone Broth:

Ingredients:

2–3 pounds chicken carcass, neck, and feet

1/2 c. raw apple cider vinegar

4 quarts filtered water

3 celery stalks, halved

3 carrots, halved

2 onions, quartered

A handful of fresh parsley (wait until last ten minutes to add this)

Sea salt

Pepper

Directions:

1. Place bones in an Instant Pot or a Crock-Pot, add apple cider vinegar and water, and let the mixture sit for 1 hour so the vinegar can leach the minerals out of the bones.

2. Add more water, if needed, to cover the bones.

3. Add the vegetables bring to a boil, skim the scum from the top, and discard.

4. Reduce to a low simmer, cover, and cook for 24–72 hours. (If you're not comfortable leaving the pot to simmer overnight, turn off the heat and let it sit overnight, then turn it back on, and let it simmer all day the next day). If using an Instant Pot, you only have to put it on high pressure for 90 minutes.

5. During the last ten minutes of cooking, throw in a handful of fresh parsley for added flavor and minerals.

6. Let the broth cool and strain it. In addition to a strainer, I put a nylon around my strainer, so it catches everything really well, and it makes for a nice clear broth.

7. Add sea salt and pepper to taste. Drink the broth as is or store it in fridge up to 5–7 days (or freeze up to 6 months) for use in soups or stews. Enjoy!

Serving Size: 3 Quarts

---

*Oven Roasted Whole Organic Chicken
(You can make two birds for batch-cooking)

Ingredients:
Whole chicken: 3–4 pounds (neck and giblets removed)
1 Tbsp. olive oil
1 and 1/2 tsp(s) sea salt
1 tsp paprika
1 tsp black pepper
1/2 tsp chopped thyme
1/2 tsp chopped rosemary
1/2 tsp chopped sage
Fresh lemon cut into quarters (to stuff inside the bird)

Directions:

1. Preheat oven to 450 degrees.
2. Rinse chicken in water, inside and out, and pat dry.
3. Combine olive oil and spices in a small bowl (depending on the size of your bird(s), you may add more if needed.)
4. Rub the spice mixture on top of and around the chicken, and then inside (under the skin) as well.
5. Place chicken breast side up on roasting pan.
6. Place lemon inside the bird.
7. Place in your preheated oven, and immediately reduce heat to 375 degrees.
8. Roast chicken at approximately 20 minutes per pound or until the temperature of the breast meat reaches 165 degrees.
9. Remove chicken, and let sit for 10 minutes before serving.

Serves 2–4, depending on the weight of the chicken. I use a smaller organic chicken. Most conventional chickens will range from 5–7 lbs., yet these are not your best choice. Cook two small organic chickens instead.

---

*Paleo Shephard's Pie

Ingredients:

1–2 cauliflowers (1 is sufficient, but I like having more for leftovers)

1 lb. grass-fed ground beef

1 lb. organic pork sausage, casings removed

1 small onion, chopped

1 c. Bellini mushrooms, chopped

1 16 oz. package of Cascadian Farms Organic Mixed Vegetables

2 c. homemade beef broth or Pacific Brand Organic Beef Bone Broth

2 Tbsp. organic butter

2–3 Tbsp. of almond flour (or any other gluten-free flour)

2 Tbsp. of Coconut Oil or Avocado Oil

Salt and pepper to taste

Directions:

1. Prepare the vegetables and chicken.
    a. Place oil in a pan; sauté onions until golden.
    b. Add mushrooms; sauté for five minutes.
    c. Add mixed vegetables to pan; sauté for five minutes.
2. Meanwhile, in a separate pan, sauté the ground beef and ground sausage until cooked throughout.
3. Prepare the gravy.
    a. Pour the bone broth and butter into a small pan.
    b. Let it come to a boil.
    c. Add the flour bit by bit, using a small strainer, whisking constantly until a gravy emerges.

Season with salt and pepper.

4. Prepare the cauliflower.
    a. Cut cauliflower into florets. Steam until soft; your fork will go through with ease.
    b. Place in a bowl with 2 Tbsp. of butter.
    c. Add salt and pepper to taste.
    d. Using an emulsion blender, blend until smooth.
5. Prepare the casserole.
    a. Pour the ground meat and gravy into the pan with vegetables, and mix all together.
    b. Pour mixture into a casserole pan.
    c. Spread mashed cauliflower on top.
    d. Bake uncovered at 375 degrees for 30 minutes or until cauliflower turns slightly brown.

Serves 4–6

DESSERT

*Chocolate Chia Pudding

Ingredients:

1/4 c. chia seeds

8 oz. full-fat canned coconut milk

1 Tbsp. maple syrup

1 Tbsp. raw cacao powder

1/2 c. chopped organic strawberries or bananas (optional)

Directions:

1. Put the first four ingredients into a mason jar with a tight-fitting lid.
2. Close and shake well to combine; then store in the fridge overnight.
3. Top with fruit in the morning, and enjoy.
4. If batch cooking, place all ingredients in a large bowl, combine, place in mason jars, and store in fridge overnight.

Serves 1 (double up for next day)

Mango-Blueberry Sorbet

Ingredients:

1 bag frozen mango

1 bag frozen blueberries

1/4–1/2 c. water or apple juice

Directions:

Blend the ingredients until creamy. Scrape down sides of blender with a spatula if needed. Serve immediately, and store extra in the freezer in a freezer-safe container.

Serves 4

Baked Apples and Pears

Ingredients:

1 cut up apple

1 cut up pear

1 tsp of apple pie spice (or combine cinnamon and nutmeg)

Directions:

Place fruit on a baking dish with a little coconut oil. Sprinkle apple pie spice or cinnamon and nutmeg over the fruit.

Bake in a 350-degree oven for about 30 minutes or until the fruit is tender.

Serves 2

Chocolate Bombs

Ingredients:

1 c. raw cashews

1/4 c. cacao powder

1/4 c. raw liquid honey

1/8 c. hemp seeds

1/8 c. chia seeds

1/8 c. shredded coconut

2 Tbsp. coconut oil, gently melted

1 small pinch vanilla bean

1 pinch sea salt

Directions:

Process all dry ingredients in a food processor or Vitamix until finely ground. Add honey and oil, and process again.

1. Roll into balls by the teaspoonful. Keep in a glass container with a tight-fitting lid in your fridge for a week or in your freezer for a month.

Serves 1-2

Ginger Yams Delight

Ingredients:

2 garnet yams, scrubbed but not peeled

1/2-inch chunk fresh ginger, grated

1–2 tsp ground ginger

1 tsp ground turmeric

1/2 (14-oz.) can full-fat coconut milk

Salt and pepper to taste

Directions:

1. Preheat oven to 375 degrees.
2. Place yams on a baking sheet lined with parchment paper, and bake for about 45 minutes or until very soft to the touch.
3. When cool, squeeze yams out of their skins into a stovetop pot.
4. Heat over medium-low heat. Add fresh and ground ginger. Then add up to 1/2 can coconut milk, 2 tablespoons at a time, being sure to incorporate milk fully into the mash before adding more.
5. Season with salt and pepper to taste.

Note: You can eat the leftovers as breakfast porridge the next day. Simply reheat, add a little more coconut milk, and top with honey, cinnamon, and walnuts.

Serves 1-2

Batch Cook Your Basics

I find the Instant Pot to be the best when making these basics. It is a great investment, as it is a huge time-saver when making otherwise cumbersome meals if you're pinched for time.

Brown Rice (Instant Pot)

Ingredients:
3 c. uncooked brown rice
3 and 1/2 c. water, vegetable stock, or broth
Dash of salt

Directions:
1. Add the uncooked brown rice with water, stock, or broth, and cover. Select the MANUAL button and the lid to seal, and set to high pressure for 22 minutes. It will take about five minutes to start, and then the countdown begins. After the allowed time, Instant Pot will automatically release the pressure on its own (about 10 minutes). Remove the lid, and fluff the rice.
2. Place leftover rice in airtight containers for later use (or freeze up to three months).

Quinoa (Instant Pot)

Ingredients:
3 c. rinsed, uncooked quinoa (rinsing gets rid of bitterness; rinse until water is clear)
3 1/2 c. water, vegetable stock, or broth
Dash of salt

Directions:
1. Spray or use a brush to line Instant Pot with avocado or coconut oil, so damp quinoa doesn't stick to the bottom.

2. Add the uncooked quinoa with water, vegetable stock, or broth and cover. Select the MANUAL button and set to high-pressure for one minute. It will take about five minutes to start, and then the countdown begins. After the allowed time, Instant Pot will automatically release pressure on its own (about 10 minutes). Remove lid, and fluff quinoa.

Book, Audio, and Video Reference Guide

Unconventional Medicine:
Join the Revolution to Reinvent Healthcare, Reverse Chronic Disease,
and Create a Practice You Love by Chris Kresser

The world is facing the greatest healthcare crisis it has ever seen. Chronic disease is shortening our lifespan, destroying our quality of life, bankrupting governments, and threatening the health of future generations. Sadly, conventional medicine, with its focus on managing symptoms, has failed to address this challenge. The result is burned-out physicians, a sicker population, and a broken healthcare system. In *Unconventional Medicine*, Chris Kresser presents a plan to reverse this dangerous trend. He shows how the combination of a genetically aligned diet and lifestyle, Functional Medicine, and a lean, collaborative practice model can create a system that better serves the needs of both patients and practitioners.

Revolution Health Radio, Chris's podcast delivers cutting-edge, yet practical, information on how to prevent and reverse disease naturally. Available on iTunes.

Food: What the Heck Should I Eat? by Mark Hyman, MD

Dr. Hyman takes a close look at every food group and explains what we've gotten wrong, revealing which foods nurture our health and which pose a threat. From grains to legumes, meat to dairy, fats to artificial sweeteners, and beyond, Dr. Hyman debunks misconceptions and breaks down the fascinating science in his signature, accessible style. He also explains food's role as powerful medicine capable of reversing chronic disease and shows how our food system and policies impact the environment, the economy, social justice, and personal health, painting a holistic picture of growing, cooking, and eating food in ways that nourish our bodies and the earth while creating a healthy society.

Radical Remission: Surviving Cancer Against All Odds
by Kelly A. Turner, PhD

Dr. Kelly A. Turner, the founder of the Radical Remission Project, uncovers nine factors that can lead to a spontaneous remission from cancer—even after conventional medicine has failed.

Chris Beat Cancer by Chris Wark

At twenty-six years old, Chris Wark was diagnosed with colon cancer. He had surgery to remove a golf ball-sized tumor and a third of his colon. But after surgery, instead of the traditional chemotherapy, Chris decided to radically change his diet and lifestyle in order to promote health and healing in his body. In *Chris Beat Cancer*, he describes his healing journey, exposes the corruption and ineffectiveness of the medical and cancer industries, and shares the strategies that he and many others have used to heal cancer.

Younger: A Breakthrough Program to Reset Your Genes, Reverse Aging, and Turn Back the Clock by Sara Gottfried, MD

The scientific reality is that 90 percent of the signs of aging and disease are caused by lifestyle choices, not your genes. In other words, you have the capability to overcome and transform your genetic history and tendencies. Harvard/MIT—trained physician Sara Gottfried, MD has created a revolutionary seven-week program that empowers us to make the critical choices necessary to not just look young, but also feel young.

The Autoimmune Epidemic by Donna Jackson Nakazawa

The author provides investigative journalism that seeks the real causes for this epidemic. Her desire to find answers was fueled by her own struggle with autoimmune disease.

Against All Grain: Meals Made Simple: Gluten-free, Dairy-Free, and Paleo Recipes to Make Anytime by Danielle Walker

Preparing real foods can be time-consuming and monotonous, but Danielle brings both simplicity and creativity to the everyday meal with an enthusiasm for flavors and textures that are often lacking in easy weeknight dishes. *Meals Made Simple* includes a variety of slow cooker, one-pot, and thirty-minute meals, as well as ways to create entirely new dishes from leftovers.

Whole 30: A 30-Day Guide To Total Health and Food Freedom by Melissa Hartwig and Dallas Hartwig

The Whole 30 offers a stand-alone, step-by-step plan to break unhealthy habits, reduce cravings, improve digestion, and strengthen your immune system. The Whole 30 prepares participants for the program in five easy steps, previews a typical thirty days, teaches the basic meal preparation and cooking skills needed to succeed, and provides a month's worth of recipes designed to build confidence in the kitchen and inspire the taste buds.

Sugar Impact Diet: Drop 7 Hidden Sugars, Lose Up to 10 Pounds in Just 2 Weeks by JJ Virgin

In this groundbreaking book, *New York Times* bestselling author JJ Virgin explains the powerful concept of "sugar impact": how different sugars react differently in the body. High sugar impact foods cause weight gain, energy crashes, and inflammation. Low sugar impact foods fuel your body for prolonged energy and promotes fat-burning.

This eye-opening book pinpoints the most damaging sugars that we eat every day—without even realizing it—in common foods like skim milk, diet soda, whole-grain bread, and "healthy" sweeteners like agave.

Healing Arthritis: Your 3-Step Guide to Conquering Arthritis Naturally by Susan Blum MD

Dr. Susan Blum, a leading expert in Functional Medicine, offers a better approach to healing arthritis permanently. Her groundbreaking three-step protocol is designed to address the underlying causes of the condition and heal the body permanently by treating rheumatoid arthritis, osteoarthritis, and more—healing your gut to heal your joints and reducing inflammation without medication.

You Are the Placebo: Making Your Mind Matter by Dr. Joe Dispenza

Dr. Joe Dispenza shares numerous documented cases of those who reversed cancer, heart disease, depression, crippling arthritis, and even the tremors of Parkinson's disease by believing in a placebo. Similarly, Dr. Joe tells of how others have gotten sick and even died the victims of a hex or voodoo curse—or after being misdiagnosed with a fatal illness. Belief can be so strong that pharmaceutical companies use double- and triple-blind randomized studies to try to exclude the power of the mind over the body when evaluating new drugs.

The Biology of Belief by Bruce Lipton

Former medical school professor and research scientist Bruce H. Lipton, PhD, presents his experiments, and those of other leading-edge scientists, which examine in great detail the mechanisms by which cells receive and process information. The implications of this research radically change our understanding of life, showing that genes and DNA do not control our biology; instead, DNA is controlled by signals from outside the cell, including the energetic messages emanating from our positive and negative thoughts.

HEAL Documentary
www.healdocumentary.com/[xxv]

A documentary film that takes us on a scientific and spiritual journey, where we discover that by changing one's perceptions, beliefs, and emotions, the human body can heal itself from any disease.

The Fat-Burning Man Podcast by Abel James

The award-winning, number-one rated *Fat-Burning Man Show*, available on iTunes, helps listeners to improve their relationship with food, activity, and life by circumventing marketing myths, misinformation, and corporate scheming by eating real foods and engaging in effective, science-backed training to make you lean, healthy, and energetic.

The Doctor's Farmacy Podcast by Mark Hyman MD

Dr. Hyman offers in-depth conversations about our health, wellness, food, and politics.

Broken-Brain Docu-Series by Mark Hyman MD
brokenbrain.com/trailer/[xxxvi]

Broken Brain is a powerful documentary series that addresses the root causes of terrifying and growing epidemics that ranges from Alzheimer's, dementia, brain injuries, ADHD, autism, depression, anxiety, concussions, and everything in between.

Interconnected, The Power to Heal From Within

Interviews with seventy renowned doctors and health experts on how to heal chronic disease, sharpen your thinking, and boost your immune system when you discover how to feed, nurture, and control your gut's microbiome. A ten-disc CD set or a digital download available at *www.interconnectedseries.com/over-2/*[xxxvii].

FMTV (Food Matters www.fmtv.com/) [xxxviii]

Food Matters TV is an online-streaming channel and a great destination where you can be guaranteed to find the best health documentaries out in the world. They search the globe for the most influential and life-changing films that exist.

Food Revolution Network foodrevolution.org:[xxxix]

John Robbins was groomed to be the heir to the Baskin-Robbins empire, which was founded by his father. He had money, prestige, and security, along with an ice cream shaped swimming pool in the backyard. So, why did John walk away from a path that was practically "paved with gold and ice cream?" Because his conscience was emerging, he simply didn't want to devote his life to selling ice cream after realizing it makes people unhealthy. So, he decided to make a change and forge a new path.

Ocean Robbins was born in a log cabin built by his parents. He grew up eating food they grew on the land together. At age sixteen, he cofounded an organization called YES! (Youth for Environmental Sanity) that he directed for the next twenty years. Ocean has spoken in person to more than 200,000 people in schools, conferences, and events, and he has organized 100+ seminars and gatherings for leaders from sixty-five-plus nations. FoodRevolution.org is an online-based education and advocacy-driven organization committed to healthy, sustainable, humane, and conscious food for all.

Benefits of Working with a Health Coach

Taking the information I have presented in this book and implementing the necessary steps can seem overwhelming and confusing at first. However, given the global rates of obesity, diabetes, and other chronic diseases on the rise, we can't ignore the situation any longer. Over 65 percent of Americans are overweight, and by 2020, estimates show that half of all Americans will suffer from a *preventable* chronic disease. The United States alone spends over $2.5 trillion every year on healthcare, with a large portion of that money coming from employers' pockets for employee health insurance, medical leave, and sick days.

Chronic stress, poor dietary habits, and lack of exercise all significantly contribute to ill-health. Luckily, many of these costly, chronic ailments are avoidable with simple, preventative care.

Having a support system in place will help you effectively manage your symptoms, or even reverse them altogether. There are many new therapies available that help treat you holistically, yet you may not be aware of them. That's why hiring a health coach can be a cost-effective solution to improve your health. A health coach will help you make better food and lifestyle choices, all the while improving your physical, mental, and spiritual well-being.

The health coaching industry is gaining momentum and awareness in mainstream media and on Capitol Hill. In fact, it is currently one of the fastest-growing career paths. More and more healthcare professionals are relying on health coaches to fill the gap between the doctor and the patient. As healthcare costs rise, a health coach can step in and help you make necessary lifestyle changes that can positively impact your health in a major way.

The following list highlights the benefits of hiring a health coach to achieve your health goals:

1. **Looks at all areas of your life, in addition to your eating habits.** Health coaches are different from a nutritionist or a dietitian. They don't just give you a list of foods or specific diet recommendations. They take it a step further by talking about your "primary foods." Primary foods relate to your environment, including career, finances, physical activity, relationships, home environment, social life, spirituality, home cooking, etc.

   Is your demanding schedule stressing you out? Are you in an unhappy relationship? Do you feel as if you are burning the candle at both ends, trying to keep up? Are you not taking time to self-nurture? A health coach will survey areas where you struggle. They look to find the root cause of your health issue by taking a holistic approach and understanding the emotional, physical, behavioral, and nutritional lifestyle factors that you need to enhance overall health and well-being.

2. **A health coach does not prescribe one diet or one way of living.** Rather, they help you develop a deeper understanding of the food and lifestyle choices that work best for your body. Some common areas where they assist you include weight management, food cravings, sleep, energy, digestion, stress, and time management. A health coach empowers you to make lasting lifestyle changes, from weight management to overall wellness. They guide, mentor, and empower you to take responsibility for your health and support you in making sustainable lifestyle choices.

3. **A health coach will create a "safe" place to open and share your thoughts, worries, concerns, etc.** They establish trust through open communication and active listening without casting judgment. Your coach will hold you accountable in a supportive way. A health coach will help you establish short- and long-term goals, by continually revisiting them to keep track of progress. They help you gain clarity on ideas and ambitions and guide you in achieving them.

4. **You will establish awareness around perception and self-talk.** A health coach will help you retrain your brain to a more positive place. They work with you to establish positive self-talk (the things we tell ourselves) by identifying limiting beliefs. By becoming aware of situations where negative self-talk occurs, you can change direction toward a more empowered state.

5. **Your health coach will teach you to become your own health advocate and to understand your body's messages.** Intuition is a key factor in health, and they will show you how to use this important gift. And, when you work with a health coach, you'll gain a new awareness in the areas of your life where you previously felt stuck. You'll feel excited to put into action all the tools and information you have learned. And you won't feel the need to succumb to the next fad diet because you will have the knowledge, confidence, and self-awareness to fuel your body with nutrient-dense foods. You can make it a lifestyle!

Making these lifestyle changes will help you to understand that when we can become present to what is not working and shift that awareness to find what is working, transformation takes place. We inherently want to take care of ourselves, feed our body with whole foods nutrition, and take time to rest and restore and allow more joy into our life.

As a health coach, I want to empower you to make informed choices. To find out more about working with me, or if you're interested in learning more about my online group coaching programs, visit my website *www.donnamarkussen.com/contact*. I look forward to hearing from you!

About the Author

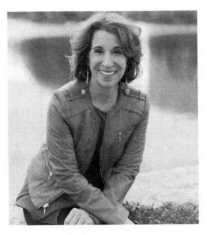

*"I went from living with chronic neck, shoulder, and back pain,
a breast cancer diagnosis at age forty-four, and an autoimmune
disease diagnosis that nearly brought me to my knees to living
a healthy, vibrant life without the use of medications.
Now I want to help you reverse disease and age fearlessly!"*
— Donna Markussen

Certified holistic health coach Donna Markussen is a wife, mother of two fabulous adult boys, and author of the books *Finding My Way: Facing My Journey with Courage* and *Finding My Way: Notes of Inspiration*.

She also is a noted in demand keynote speaker and a breast cancer survivor who has helped thousands of women make transformative changes to their mind, body, and soul.

Donna understands firsthand the confusion and fear of living with a frightening health diagnosis when you don't know which step is the right one to take on your journey back to good health. She knows exactly how confusing it can be to navigate your way around our Western medical model, but she's also an expert on how to maneuver out of the madness.

Donna knows that when you receive a debilitating diagnosis, the first thing you feel is fear. Fear of the unknown. Fear that you may have to live with your condition. And fear that you'll never be able to enjoy your kids or grandchildren again.

As a holistic health coach, Donna uses an arsenal of coaching tools, paired with her natural communication skills, to help her clients make the diet, lifestyle, and behavior changes that are the key to reversing chronic disease. And instead of just treating symptoms, Donna teaches the awareness of the Functional Medicine approach that addresses the underlying root cause of disease.

She believes that food is the best medicine and that we must address those negative influences in our lives that may be harming our health. Self-awareness and understanding our body's symptoms are key ingredients in finding your own health.

Her goal is to provide training, education, and information through one-on-one coaching, group programs, and community and corporate wellness programs, empowering others to take back control of their bodies and minds to live long, healthy lives.

To learn more about Donna's programs, please visit
www.DonnaMarkussen.com
www.facebook.com/donnamarkussen2016/
twitter.com/dmarkussen
www.instagram.com/donnamarkussen/
www.linkedin.com/in/dmarkussen/

Acknowledgments

Thank you to my editor, Cynde Christie. You have worked so diligently on my behalf, shaping my mountain of blogs and articles into a readable manuscript while always embracing my new ideas, changes in the format, and new insights, and not making me feel guilty.

Thank you, Casey Demchak, my copywriter, for developing my core marketing message platform and capturing the essence of this book so profoundly.

Thank you, Jen Zelinger, for your patience with the multiple revisions you endured working on the manuscript. Your efforts revealed a clear, well-organized product.

Thank you, Nick Zelinger, for honoring my creative ideas for the cover and for diligently working on formatting the book to be ready for publication.

Thank you to my team of beta readers: Alice Griffin, Anne Lyon, Diane McKenzie, Fran Goldstein, Gretel Underwood, Lisa Keohane, Marianne Wronka, Mary Sloane, Robin Uglietto, Sue Ganter, and Tina Olson. Each of you selflessly took time to review the raw manuscript and then provide honest feedback. This act of service enabled me to find the areas that needed more clarity, organization, and detail. Thank you!

Index

Endnotes

[i] Anand, Preetha, Ajaikumar B Kunnumakkara, Chitra Sundaram, Kuzhuvelil B Harikumar, Sheeja T Tharakan, Oiki S Lai, Bokyung Sung, and Bharat B Aggarwal. 2008. "Cancer Is a Preventable Disease That Requires Major Lifestyle Changes." Pharmaceutical Research. Springer US. September 2008. *https://www.ncbi.nlm.nih.gov/pmc/articles/PMC2515569/.*

[ii] *https://healdocumentary.com*

[iii] *https://www.nap.edu/catalog/13497/us-health-in-international-perspective-shorter-lives-poorer-health*

[iv] *https://www.cdc.gov/chronicdisease/about/costs/index.htm*

[v] *https://www.livescience.com/37703-epigenetics.html*

[vi] *https://www.ifm.org*

[vii] *https://www.cancer.gov/about-cancer/causes-prevention/risk/age*

[viii] *https://www.cdc.gov/heartdisease/facts.htm*

[ix] *https://www.ncbi.nlm.nih.gov/pmc/articles/PMC4099943/*

[x] *https://www.niehs.nih.gov/health/materials/autoimmune_diseases_508.pdf*

[xi] *https://www.cdc.gov/nchs/fastats/obesity-overweight.htm*

[xii] *https://www.health.harvard.edu/blog/statin-use-is-up-cholesterol-levels-are-down-are-americans-hearts-benefiting-201104151518*

[xiii] *https://doi.org/10.1038/sj.bjc.6604684*

[xiv] *https://bit.ly/2EF9B9J*

[xv] *https://abcnews.go.com/Technology/story?id=8322077&page=1*

[xvi] *https://www.nurseshealthstudy.org/sites/default/files/pdfs/n2011.pdf*

[xvii] *https://www.ncbi.nlm.nih.gov/pubmed/24833586*

[xviii] *http://med.stanford.edu/news/all-news/2009/02/new-evidence-of-hormone-therapy-causing-breast-cancer-stanford-professor-says.html*

[xix] *www.ifm.org*

[xx] *www.naturopathic.org*

[xxi] *https://www.ncbi.nlm.nih.gov/pubmed/12696080*

[xxii] Dry Farm Wines @ *https://www.dryfarmwines.com*

[xxiii] *https://www.ncbi.nlm.nih.gov/pubmed/28174772*

[xxiv] *https://www.ncbi.nlm.nih.gov/pubmed/23949208*

[xxv] *http://seafood.edf.org/guide/best/healthy*

[xxvi] *www.GrassLandBeef.com*

[xxvii] *http://seafood.edf.org/guide/best/healthy*

[xxviii] *https://www.ewg.org/tapwater*

[xxix] *https://www.thinkdirtyapp.com/*

[xxx] *https://www.ewg.org/*

[xxxi] *https://cspinet.org/new/201006291.html*

[xxxii] *https://www.butcherbox.com*

[xxxiii] *https://waldenlocalmeat.com/what-is-a-share/*

[xxxiv] *http://www.wisechoicemarket.com/*

[xxv] *http://www.healdocumentary.com/*

[xxxvi] *https://brokenbrain.com/trailer/*

[xxxvii] *https://www.interconnectedseries.com/over-2/*

[xxxviii] *https://www.fmtv.com/*

[xxxix] *https://foodrevolution.org*

Made in the USA
Lexington, KY
27 October 2019